Hĸ. Bauer
Color Atlas of Colposcopy
3rd edition

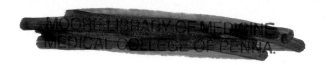

Color Atlas of Colposcopy

by

Hanskurt Bauer, M.D.
Specialist in Gynecology and Obstetrics,
Wiesbaden, West Germany

3rd revised and expanded edition

including 314 illustrations, 156 in color

IGAKU-SHOIN   New York • Tokyo

HANSKURT BAUER, M.D.
Specialist in Gynecology and Obstetrics
Biebricher Allee 135
D-6200 Wiesbaden, West Germany

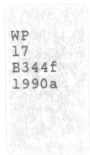
Published and distributed by

IGAKU-SHOIN Ltd.,
5-24-3 Hongo, Bunkyo-ku, Tokyo

IGAKU-SHOIN Medical Publishers, Inc.
1140 Avenue of the Americas, New York, N. Y. 10036

This book is an authorized translation from the third German edition published and copyright © 1989, 1981 and 1976 by F. K. Schattauer Verlagsgesellschaft mbH, Lenzhalde 3, D-7000 Stuttgart 1, Germany. Title of the German edition: Farbatlas der Kolposkopie. ISBN 3-7945-1257-X

Library of Congress Cataloging-in-Publication Data

Bauer, Hanskurt.
  Color atlas of colposcopy.

  Translation of: Farbatlas der Kolposkopie.
  Includes bibliographical references and index.
  1. Colposcopy—Atlases. I. Title.
RG107.5.06B3813 1990   618.1'07545   90-4868

ISBN 0-89640-182-0 (New York)

ISBN 4-260-14182-1 (Tokyo)

Printed in Germany

10 9 8 7 6 5 4 3 2 1

for my wife Christel

Preface to the Third Edition

Since the first edition of this atlas was published in 1976, colposcopy has experienced a tremendous upsurge not only in German-speaking countries but worldwide as well. The second edition also received positive acknowledgment from my colleagues, leading to this third edition. Even today, however, there is a great backlog in learning this very important method of clinical examination. Consequently, the layout of the atlas remains unchanged to serve as an introduction to this examining method. Emphasis is again placed on the figures, each of which is accompanied by a short descriptive text. Numerous new developments have necessitated a complete revision, particularly in replacing old figures with newer, more impressive ones. Enlargements of the photographs, where required, are made directly from color slides (half Leica format – 18 × 24 mm) to 7.5 cm.

A special section deals extensively with viral diseases, a topic of great current relevance. Several changes have been made in the colposcopic nomenclature.

This edition of the atlas features a much more comprehensive text and more illustrations in order to be of greater use to the reader. Consequently, a large selection of colposcopic findings found in everyday practice is available.

My thanks go out to my colleague, Dr. IRENE SIMKO, who supplied me with cases out of her practice for photodocumentation. I also wish to express special thanks to my coworker, Mrs. IRMGARD PLATTE, who, as in earlier editions, diligently and accurately typed the entire text.

At this time, I would like to again thank the Schattauer-Verlag for their dependable and generous support. My thanks are especially directed to Mr. BERGEMANN, Professor Dr. Dr. h. c. P. MATIS and Mr. KRAUSE. Mr. BÜRSCHGENS drew the illustrations in the expected excellent manner, for which I would also like to extend my gratitude.

HANSKURT BAUER

Preface to the Second Edition

Worldwide interest has been shown in the **Color Atlas of Colposcopy** to the extent that it is now published in six languages. Colposcopy has progressed and spread since the appearance of the first edition. It is an indispensable clinical examining method and should be part of every thorough clinical examination. This has been taken into consideration in the preparation of this edition. New color colpophotographs have been added and a number of figures replaced. The reader is presented an even greater and more complete selection of colposcopic findings. Colposcopic nomenclature has been updated to the latest standard.

For the first time the reader has the opportunity to order a set of color stereo slides with a viewer that complements the figures in the atlas. This allows a threedimensional viewing of the colposcopic findings – as if examining the patient firsthand. The stereo slides are without an accompanying text and therefore only of use in conjunction with the atlas.

Since the death of my esteemed teacher, Professor Dr. H. WURM, I have consulted with Professor Dr. REMMELE, Director of the Pathological Institute of the Wiesbaden City Clinic, and his head physician, Professor Dr. BETTENDORF, on histological matters. I would like to thank them for their suggestions. My thanks also go out to Professor Dr. GRIMMER, Director of the Wiesbaden City Dermatological Clinic, for his assistance in the diagnosis of vulval diseases. My colleague Dr. SIMKO was kind enough to place photographs of several cases from her practice at our disposal.

After the death of Mr. P. HAMMESFAHR, Mr. H. TSCHÖRNER drew the illustrations for the figures new to this edition. I thank him for his valuable assistance. During the printing, Mr. FRITZ LEISEGANG, Berlin, passed away. His inventive ideas led among other things to the development of the stereo camera colposcope with which I work. Color stereophotography of colposcopic findings was his lifework. It will be continued in this atlas.

Wiesbaden, Spring 1981   HANSKURT BAUER

Contents

1: Development and Significance of Colposcopy

The first colposcope was designed in 1925 by HANS HINSELMANN of Hamburg (Fig. 1.1). His ingenious idea of constructing an instrument that allows the uterine cervix, the vagina, and the vulva to be inspected under optimal illumination and with a certain degree of magnification led to the current worldwide application of this technique.

A number of authors worldwide consider that this method allows the clinician a unique opportunity to participate actively in the timely diagnosis of cervical carcinoma. In addition to early detection of cervical carcinoma and its precursors, colposcopy is particularly useful in differential diagnosis of the majority of benign cervical, vaginal, and vulval lesions, thus eliminating the need for other diagnostic procedures. Minute tissue defects such as small erosions, tiny tumors, or micro-hemorrhages within the cervical, vaginal, and vulval epithelium are frequently detectable only through optical magnification. Consequently, colposcopy has become an indispensable tool for gynecologic examination. Even sceptical colleagues soon acknowledge that lesions of the lower genital tract can be much better identified and distinguished with an optical instrument and adequate light source than by the unassisted eye.

In VEIT/STOECKEL's textbook of gynecology, HINSELMANN emphasized the clinical importance of his first colposcope by saying: "In order to demarcate the diagnosis between epithelial changes and neoplasia with certainty, it became necessary to intensify the illumination and to enlarge the image without loss of three-dimensional vision." For that purpose he employed the Leitz dissection magnifier with a solid tripod (Fig. 1.2).

Using the focal length of 14 cm and a magnification of × 10 the cervix can be inspected without clamping or otherwise touching it, and with a minimum of discomfort to the patient. With regard to practical application, HINSELMANN designed an improved version of his first colposcope for scientific purposes (Fig. 1.3), making it

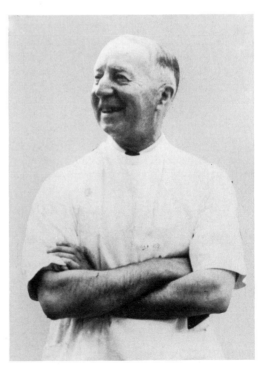

Fig. 1.1. HANS HINSELMANN (born August 6, 1884, died August 18, 1959). This picture was taken during a visit to Rio de Janeiro, South America. (This print was kindly given to me by his son, DR. HINSELMANN.)

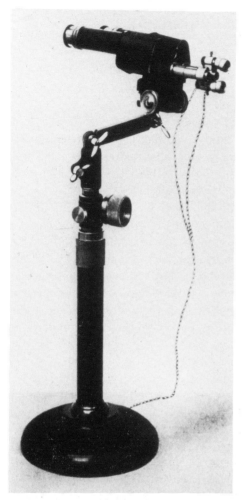

Fig. 1.2. Leitz dissection magnifier equipped for binocular inspection and with built-in light source (focal length 14 cm, magnification ×3, 5, 7 and 10.5).

possible to observe the cervix with a bright white light under even higher magnification.

In his many publications HINSELMANN frequently emphasized the ability of colposcopy to differentiate, in living tissue, between carcinomatous and other epithelial lesions that had previously caused diagnostic difficulties. During repeated visits to South America, HINSELMANN found that appreciation of his method was greater there than in Germany. Societies for cer-

vical pathology and colpomicroscopy were founded not only in Brazil but also in Argentina.

Colposcopy is also done in other South American countries, for example, in Colombia. In Bogota I had the opportunity to perform colposcopy in several clinics and was invited by the Colombian Society for Colposcopy and Cervical Pathology to hold lectures and seminars.

In the United States the development of colposcopy began in 1963 with the founding of a society. Since then a continual upward development is evident, with numerous seminars and workshops being held throughout the country. The journal *The Colposcopist* regularly provides society members with new developments and education on the subject of colposcopy.

In the meantime the use of colposcopy has spread worldwide. A world organization was founded in Mar del Plata, Argentina, in 1972. I personally had the honor to be present in my function as chairman of the German study association Cervix Uteri. The meeting was well attended, with nearly 1000 participants. Six World Congresses have since been held: in Europe (Graz, Austria, and London, England), in South America (Mar del Plata, Argentina), in the United States (Orlando, Florida), and in Japan (Tokyo).

According to the latest figures, the International Society for Cervical Pathology and Colposcopy is now the representative organization for 21 national societies.

In the German Democratic Republic as in most Eastern European countries, colposcopy is a well-established part of the clinical examination both for early detection of carcinoma and routine gynecological examination. Here credit must be given to GANSE, a student of HINSELMANN, whose personality and teamwork with his colleagues have positively influenced the advancement of colposcopy. In 1987 I had the pleasure of lecturing on colposcopy in Dresden at the gynecological clinic of the Medical Academy Carl-Gustav-Carus, where GANSE had worked. That same year I also lectured at the University Gynecological Clinic in Halle. Previously I had been a guest at university gynecological clinics in Leipzig and Rostock.

LANE wrote the first textbook on colposcopy in a Slavic language (Czechoslovakian and Russian) in 1956. Over the years as chairman of the study association Cervix Uteri, now the Study Association of Cervical Pathology and Colposcopy, I have always considered it important to keep in contact with the colleagues from Eastern European countries. I have been invited to Hungary several times to lecture at several university gynecological clinics, and I have even participated in a congress in Bulgaria. My relationship with the gynecological clinic of the Medical Academy in Krakow, Poland, is especially friendly. Under the chairmanship of J. MADEJ, regular workshops and continuing education programs are held in which I take part.

Colposcopy is well recognized outside of Germany in the remaining European countries, especially in Switzerland and Austria. Outstanding scientists have con-

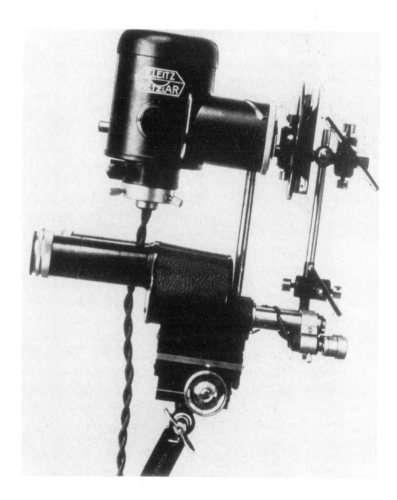

Fig. 1.3. Colposcope for scientific investigation with an illumination attachment (top) and binocular tube. Leitz dissection magnifier with ×10, 20, 30 and 40 magnification.

tributed to its propagation – above all WESPI in Switzerland, who first described stereocolposcopy.

Close scientific and personal relations have also developed with various university gynecological clinics in South Africa. In 1988 I took part in the 24th Workshop of the South African Society of Obstetrics and Gynecology. Further lectures were held in Johannesburg, Durban, Pretoria, and Cape Town. Colposcopy is particularly intensively pursued at the Stellenbosch university gynecological clinic at Tygerberg Hospital in Cape Town.

Strangely enough, although developed in Germany, colposcopy established itself only slowly in its country of origin. The reasons are complex. Originally the fault may have lain with HINSELMANN himself, because he directed the method solely toward the diagnosis of early carcinoma and because he tried to enforce his own terminology. His insistence that leukoplakia is always a carcinomatous precursor gained him many opponents. His failure to obtain a professorial chair certainly delayed the expansion of colposcopy.

In the intervening years the techniques of cytologic examination, originating in America, have prevailed. Interpreting and recording cytologic findings became relatively easy. Colposcopy inevitably lagged behind because it required a considerable amount of experience and because adequate forms of colposcopic documentation were not available until recently. As late as 1974, MESTWERDT and WESPI stated that the teaching of colposcopy, unlike the teaching of cytology, required the presence of a patient – one could not simply set up some 40 microscopes with the appropriate cytological slides. Fortunately, we are now able to train groups of 40 or more persons simultaneously without a patient. Each participant receives a stereo slide viewer and a series of color stereo slides on all relevant colposcopic situations. The quality of these slide copies is excellent and almost reproduces the real image as seen at the actual examination of the patient. (This technique is further described and illustrated in Chapter 2.)

The development and propagation of colposcopy has made great progress. A number of university gynecological clinics in the Federal Republic of Germany have established dysplasia consultations to which patients with suspicious or positive cytologic smears (Pap test) are referred to undergo colposcopy. Although this is not an ideal solution – ideal would be that *every thorough examination include colposcopy* – progress has been made. Nevertheless, the teaching of colposcopy is still much neglected, whereas cytology is an established part of the curriculum in postgraduate education.

In 1968 an international symposium was held in Hamburg under the guidance of WESPI and of MESTWERDT, a student of HINSELMANN, who until his death in December 1979 was probably the best known authority on the subject. Researchers and clinicians from all over the world attended to discuss atypical alterations of the cervical epithelium. At that time it was unequivocally stated that for the early detection of cervical malignancy, colposcopy and cytology should be employed together for optimum and accurate diagnosis. This opinion is as valid today as it was then. In 1972 the study association Cervix Uteri was founded. Private practitioners, clinicians, and researchers convened to discuss the physiology and pathology of the uterine cervix as well as changes of the vagina and vulva. A systematic program for continuing education in colposcopy and gynecological cytology was set up.

The study association has since grown to 250 members from ten countries and is still affiliated with the German Society of Gynecology and Obstetrics. The main field of activity is cervical pathology and colposcopy, but related topics are also pursued. Nine workshops with international participation have been held to date. In 1986 M. HILGARTH took charge of the study association, which altered its name to Association for the Study of Cervical Pathology and Colposcopy to conform internationally.

A number of additional meetings and publications have demonstrated the importance of colposcopy along with the cytologic smear (Papanicolaou test) for timely detection of early stages of cervical carcinoma and its precursors. The 95 to 99% accuracy formerly attributed to the Pap test has been found much too high. Although an accuracy of approximately 80% in detecting precursors and early stage carcinoma is currently assumed, a study of 923 cases from 34 gynecologic practices and clinics in which early stage carcinoma or precursors were histologically proven, the accuracy rate was found to be 75.6%. At the 43rd meeting of the German Society of Gynecology and Obstetrics in Hamburg in 1980, experts who participated in a roundtable discussion on this subject stated that:

Colposcopy should be part of every thorough gynecologic examination.

Colposcopy is capable of improving the quality of cervical smears, and therefore in current gynecologic practice no cervical smear should be taken except under colposcopic control.

Photodocumentation of colposcopic findings definitely enhances diagnosis; among its uses are followup of abnormal findings and therapeutic methods.

Current techniques of photodocumentation present no technical problems and are financially affordable.

Directed (punch) biopsy under colposcopic observation is a proven, accurate diagnostic method whereby tissue is excised from the colposcopically most suspicious area of the external cervix.

This worldwide progress in the adoption of colposcopy for the benefit of our patients is an indication of its enormous value as a clinical evaluation method. Noticeable progress is finally also being made in the Federal Republic of Germany, the country in which colposcopy originated. Every prospective gynecologist and obstetrician should have command of the rudiments of colposcopy and cytology. This in turn stresses the importance of teaching and continuing education. The positive development in university and other gynecologic clinics is a sign that the Association for the Study of Cervical Pathology and Colposcopy was not founded in vain. Numerous continuing education courses in colposcopy repeatedly impress upon colleagues the significance of colposcopy in daily practice. As already stated, HINSELMANN had already recognized the importance of colposcopy over 60 years ago, not only for the early detection of malignant cervical precursors but also for differentiation between benign cervical lesions. This second potential renders the technique particularly valuable in daily practice, and nobody who is familiar with the use of colposcopy would do a gynecologic examination without it. Practitioners who do colposcopy routinely are well aware that genuine malignant precursors are rare and that most findings are epithelial changes of a benign nature.

2: Colposcopic Technique

2.1 Instruments

A binocular instrument specifically is recommended, because monocular colposcopes lack stereoscopic three-dimensional vision, which is particularly important. A colposcope used in the daily routine should be easily manageable and requires a high quality binocular lens and a good light source. The magnifying power should be ×10 to ×15, the optimum range for identifying epithelial and vascular changes on the cervical, vaginal, and vulval surfaces.

The major German manufacturers of colposcopes, to my knowledge, are Leisegang and Zeiss. They produce technically excellent instruments for which photographic attachments are available. My personal experience of more than 35 years was first gained with the Zeiss colposcope and later with the Möller colposcope, which is no longer made. For 21 years now I have used the stereocamera colposcope from Leisegang and will therefore describe it first.

2.1.1 Leisegang Stereocamera Colposcopes

Since in my opinion the future of practical colposcopy lies in the documentation of colposcopic findings, I am beginning with the description of the instrument that I use daily and that has given me the best photographic results. For private practice the stereocamera colposcope model IIIBD appears to be particularly suitable because even the nontechnically minded can take photographs without difficulty.

My previous experience with colpophotography was unfortunately not always the best, and I was surprised to see how easy it is to photograph with this apparatus. The basic principle is that the examiner be able to produce a color picture of colposcopic observations with the minimum of expense, no unnecessary delay, and no extra discomfort to the patient. The undisturbed evaluation of the slides and comparison with previous findings can be carried out later with the help of a special stereoscopic viewer. Since the stereoslides are usually framed by the processing laboratory, no additional work is involved.

The colposcope model IIIBD (Fig. 2.1) has a binocular lens system for stereoscopic inspection. At a working distance of 24 or 30 cm, depending on preference, magnifications of ×7.5, ×15, or ×30 are possible. Photography, however, is only possible at ×15. The infinitely variable regulation of the halogen lamp permits the illuminated area to exactly match the viewing field (×7.5 magnification) to be examined. A laterally attached handle permits focusing and a thorough search of the cervical surface. The colposcope is further equipped with an electronic flash. During exposure, the flash operates through the light source passage by means of a moving mirror so that the reflections during inspection and flash photography cover the same fields, and consequently the nonreflecting areas in the photographs are the same as when directly viewed. The very short exposure time of 1/800 prevents taking blurred pictures. By clos-

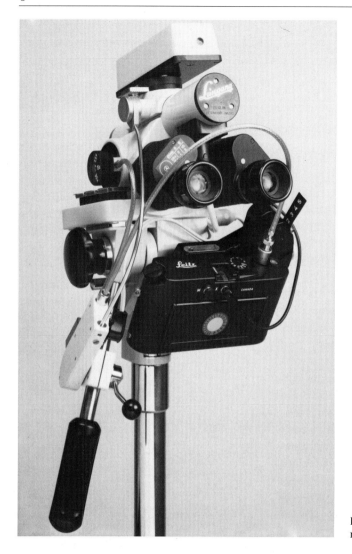

Fig. 2.1. Stereocamera   colposcope
model IIIBD from Leisegang, Berlin.

ing the aperture considerably, it is possible to obtain prints with excellent depth
of field. A small lever above the focusing handle operates the camera, the electronic flash, and the mirror reflectors for
switching from illumination lighting over
to electronic flash. Thus, an essential
requirement is fulfilled: When focusing
the image during colposcopy, the examiner automatically receives a sharp picture.
A labeled film marker containing the film
number, patient's name and date of the
examination is simultaneously exposed
on the same negative for later identification.

New instruments are now being offered
with cold light illumination. The darker
×30 magnification is thereby automatically adjusted to the same illumination
level that is observed with the ×15 magnification. The illuminated area is also adjusted to correspond with the magnification used.

The choice of film is of course very important. At present the color daylight reversal
film from both Agfa and Kodak (21 DIN =

100 ASA) can be recommended. They are of equally good quality. Excellent duplicates can be made from the stereo slides for teaching purposes.

The above-mentioned stereocamera colposcope is also obtainable without photographic accessories, and it can be refitted as a Polaroid camera colposcope. This so-called "stereo-print-camera-colposcope" also takes three-dimensional photos which can be viewed with a special slide viewer provided by Leisegang. The colposcope can also be fitted to take normal 24×36 mm color pictures, but there are definite advantages to Polaroid prints, for example, when an immediate picture is demanded. This can be the case in hospitals, polyclinics, or private practices in which a patient is regularly examined. The colpophotographs can be immediately put in the patient's records. Of course, the quality of Polaroid pictures is poorer than that of stereo slides and they are much more expensive.

Other simpler colposcopes without photographic attachments are also manufactured, eg, the standard colposcope I (Fig. 2.2). The model ID and the cold light colposcope (Fig. 2.3) have magnifications of ×7.5, ×15, and ×30. A regular feature is the already mentioned light adaptability mechanism and a higher positioned eyepiece.

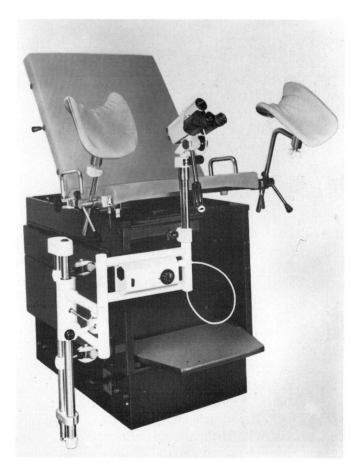

Fig. 2.2. Standard Leisegang colposcope model I with swivel arm.

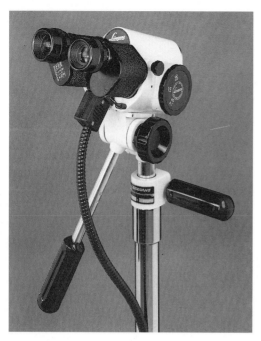

Fig. 2.3. Leisegang cold light colposcope model IDF

All standard colposcopes delivered over the last decades can be adapted for photography, though not for stereophotography. The quality of the two-dimensional pictures is reputedly good, although I have no personal experience to report on. Any camera with interchangeable lenses can be used; the photoadapter is permanently attached to the colposcope, and the camera can be detached in a single step. All Leisegang colposcopes are fitted with a green filter and have a swivel or horizontal folding arm for mounting on the examining chair. The instruments are simple to use and not time consuming. The new models are also equipped with a laser adapter.

In addition to the stereocamera colposcope model IIIBD, a video attachment can be obtained. It consists of an adapter provided by Leisegang plus a small portable videocamera that can be quickly attached to the colposcope on the left side

(Fig. 2.4). A monitor can be mounted on the wall or suspended from the ceiling, allowing the patient to follow the examination along with the physician. For cases in which treatment is required or a diagnosis needs clarification, the physician is better able to explain the situation to the patient. Since in most cases the colposcopic finding is normal, the visual confirmation has a reassuring effect on the patient. In my experience, patients react very positively toward this kind of clarification. Photodocumentation should not be neglected, however, because it is valuable in forensic questions and in scientific research.

The colposcope can also be used for continuing education. Monitors with loudspeakers can be set up, and the examiner can use a microphone to convey the colposcopic findings directly to course participants without disturbing the patient. Video tapes can also be made for teaching purposes.

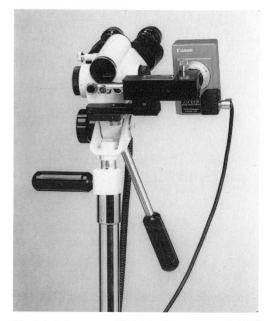

Fig. 2.4. Leisegang cold light colposcope model IDF with adapter and videocamera.

2.1.2 Zeiss Colposcopes

Zeiss (Oberkochen) has been manufacturing colposcopes for nearly 50 years. Their optics are excellent, although the initial investment for a Zeiss colposcope is considerably higher than for instruments from other manufacturers. The choice of various magnifications (up to ×40) is doubtless advantageous for the physician. A lower magnification can be used to gain a general impression, and unclear or suspicious areas can then be studied more carefully at a higher magnification at which details are more easily recognized. Higher magnifications are especially important for research and continuing education, whereas ×12 to ×15 magnifications are generally satisfactory for routine use in daily practice.

Taking photographs was formerly extremely complicated and difficult as my own experiences confirm. Photographic techniques have improved greatly over the years, however. An additional apparatus is available for stereophotography, which according to Zeiss is easy to use. I have had no personal experience with it. The Model I colposcope shown in Fig. 2.5 has a rotational disk with five magnifications and is provided with manual fine adjustment. The light source is incorporated into the swivel arm. Photographic attachments (Polaroid or miniature camera) can be installed. The flash attachment 240 available for this purpose offers a higher flash density and mirror bundling through a coaxial flash and reflection arm located in front of the convex lens (Fig. 2.6).

The colposcope Model 99 is a small, extremely easy to handle examination instrument (Fig. 2.7). The 100-watt halogen lamp can be regulated and is integrated together with the electric cord in the swivel arm. A green filter can be

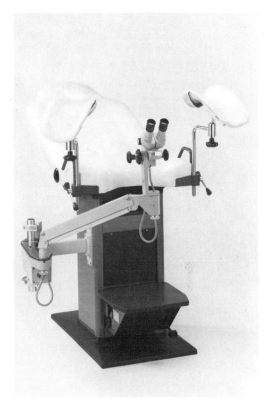

Fig. 2.5. Zeiss colposcope model I with the electric cord integrated into the swivel arm mounted on the examining chair.

folded in for greater contrast. Three different magnifications – ×8, ×12, and ×20 – can be engaged by rotating the magnifying disk. A stereobase of 16 mm permits examination with the smallest speculum. A folding arm with an elastic force balance allows the speculum to be brought effortlessly into any position.

2.1.3 Other Colposcopes

Because of its traditions, I would briefly like to describe the colposcope manufactured by Möller (Wedel) in collaboration with HINSELMANN.

Unfortunately, Möller no longer makes colposcopes. I personally used the standard model with ×10 and ×20 magnification and photoattachment for 12 years. I

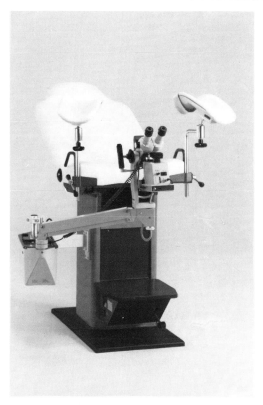

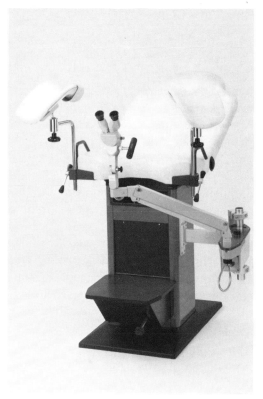

Fig. 2.6. Photocolposcope with Polaroid camera CB 71 and computerized flash.

Fig. 2.7. Zeiss colposcope model 99 with the electric cord integrated into the swivel arm.

can most assuredly attest to the excellence of the optical equipment. However, photography was possible only by raising the voltage to achieve an increased light intensity, which was not an ideal solution. Further, only flat film photography was possible. Like all models marketed at the time, the colposcope was equipped with a swivel arm that could be attached to the examining chair. Möller also manufactured a so-called special colposcope with a ×12 magnification. The other technical details were the same as in the standard model.

2.1.4 Kaps Colposcopes

The Karl Kaps Company (Asslar-Wetzlar) manufactures several colposcopes. Their models are similar to those produced by Leisegang and Zeiss. The model SOM5 can be delivered with a mobile tripod or a double swivel arm attachment. It is a stereomicroscope with a working distance of 25 cm and is equipped with a halogen or cold light lamp. Magnification is ×10. The instrument can also be supplied with a three-phase magnification rotating disk (up to ×20.5 magnification). A second model is the KP 2000S. This colposcope can also be delivered with a swivel arm (for attachment to the examining chair). Built-in photographic equipment is also available. By exchanging lenses, a magnification of ×40 can be reached (×16 magnification is standard equipment). The light source is a halogen lamp, and a green filter can be folded in.

2.1.5 The Krombach Colposcope

The firm of Krombach and Son (Wetzlar) produces a colposcope with halogen lighting and interchangeable green and blue filters. The instrument can be delivered either with a mobile stand or a double swivel arm. Wall or ceiling attachment is also possible. Here, too, the ocular lenses have to be exchanged when a different magnification is desired. This is a definite disadvantage in private practice. Assuming the average working distance is 25 cm, with an ×8 ocular lens the magnification is ×13.

Magnifications up to ×32 are possible. A second tube can be attached to permit simultaneous inspection by another person. Camera, film, or video attachments can be mounted with just a few minor adjustments, allowing the observed findings to be simultaneously recorded for teaching and documentation. I have had no personal experience with this colposcope.

Finally, the Jenoptic colposcope (Jena) is manufactured in the German Democratic Republic. According to my information, the company produces two models – the 111 and 121. The standard model 111, for routine examinations, has a permanent magnification of only ×12.5. A built-in switch in the handle permits one-handed operation of the colposcope. A halogen lamp serves as the light source. The model 121 is a variation of the 111 model with a five-phase (×4 to ×40) magnification alternator. The colposcope can be retrofitted as a photocolposcope with electronic flash.

2.1.6 Colposcopes of Non-German Manufacture

At the third World Congress for Cervical Pathology and Colposcopy 1978 in Orlando, Florida, I was first introduced to the Olympus Colposcope. I tested it for a while and found the optics very good. The 100-watt halogen lamp allows photographing without a flash. The model I tested had a ×6 to ×20 zoom magnification with infinitely variable regulation. Photographs can be taken at all magnifications. Photodocumentation is in the form of two-dimensional slides or prints. A Polaroid camera adapter is available.

The recording of the individual data for photodocumentation is not satisfactory in this model, however. The adjustment knobs on the back of the camera must be reset after each picture is taken. The colposcope is also equipped with a green filter. The somewhat too short 22-cm working distance can be increased to 30 cm by inserting a special attachment, but this reduces the magnification by approximately 25%.

Other Japanese colposcopes are built by Toitu (Tokyo) and Inami (Tokyo). Both instruments can also be obtained with photographic equipment. Several magnifications are possible, and the colposcopes are fitted with halogen lamps. The Toitu colposcope has a working distance of 22 cm, the Inami 30 cm. A third Japanese colposcope is the Monarch binocular stereocolposcope manufactured by the Green Medix Corporation (Tokyo). It has a ×15 magnification and a much too short working distance of 20 cm. With these instruments I also have no personal experience.

The excellent Leisegang and Zeiss colposcopes are strongly represented on the American market. There is also the Frigitronics 280 model made by Connecticut Incorporated of Shelton, Connecticut. It has a working distance of 25 cm. Magnifications of ×8 to ×32 can be achieved by changing the ocular lenses. Photographic equipment can be fitted on later. I am not aware of any other American - colposcopes.

For the sake of completeness I would like to mention the cervicograph developed by STAFL of Milwaukee, Wisconsin, in 1981. The instrument consists of a 100-mm macrolens with a 35-mm camera attached via a 50-mm intermediary piece. The light source (electronic flash) is located between the lens and the vaginal speculum. A very short exposure time is possible because of the extremely high flash intensity. Taking blurred pictures is therefore impossible, but the circular flash clearly causes more irritating light reflections. The cervicograph slide is projected on a screen, 10 feet or greater in width, and observed from a distance of 3 feet. In my opinion, the enlargement of the projected slide is comparable to a direct visual colposcopic magnification of 1:16. The technique differs from colposcopic photodocumentation in that a special camera takes the picture directly at the cervix.

An experienced examiner can take excellent photographs. O. BAADER, now deceased, took similarly excellent photos years ago with a Rolleiflex. The cervicograph was developed as a screening instrument and also intended for use by inexperienced technicians and physicians with relatively little experience. It is my opinion, however, that an inexperienced examiner is not likely to be capable of taking good colposcopic pictures. Obtaining a useful image begins with the proper focusing of the cervix and continues with the necessary photographic preparations, swabbing the cervix, performing the acetic acid test, and so on. All these techniques require experience.

2.2 Examining Procedure

2.2.1 Colposcopic Technique

A colposcopic examination should be performed at every gynecologic examination. A macroscopic inspection on the vulva, vagina, and cervix should first be performed. Two ordinary specula or a self-retaining speculum of the Cusco type may be used according to the custom of the examiner. Employing two separate specula, an anterior and posterior blade, has in my opinion always proved to be a reliable method of examination since pathologic alterations within the vagina cannot easily be missed. I share this view with my teacher HASELHORST.

The next step is the inspection of the cervical surface through the colposcope. Removal of any interfering mucous secretion is followed by an obligatory swabbing of the cervix with 3% acetic acid. Only then is it possible to positively identify benign cervical changes, which make up over 90% of observed changes. The columnar epithelium stands out as white grapelike structures; the metaplastic epithelium of the transformation zone stains white. The white color is a vital factor in identifying atypical epithelial changes. The mechanism of the effect of acetic acid on the epithelium is not entirely understood. Apparently a swelling effect of protein precipitation is caused, whereupon acetic acid enters the epithelium. This is the case in metaplasia and dysplasia, as well as carcinomatous epithelial growth.

An instrument tray placed next to the examiner's dominant hand should include:

A container with dry cotton swabs
Long anatomic pincettes or swab-holding forceps
A wooden cotton-tipped swab stick

Two-bladed specula of different sizes
Acetic acid solution (3%)
Lugol's iodine solution
Normal saline solution
Materials required for a Papanicolaou
smear

Colposcopy can be performed even with
nulliparous women and virgins without
injury if a slender speculum is used.
A number of different endocervical specula have been recommended for inspection
of the cervical canal. My own experience
in this respect is limited, but I share the
opinion of MESTWERDT and WESPI that
cytologic smears from the endocervix are
definitely superior.
In multiparous women the lower part of
the cervical canal is easily visualized by
separating the anterior and posterior lips
of the cervix. Keeping the posterior blade
of the speculum in one hand, the colposcopist moves the colposcope in front of
the vaginal introitus and, after switching
on the light, focuses at the correct distance on the cervical surface. The assist-
ing person holds the anterior blade with
one hand, using the other free hand to
hand any required instrument to the examiner. After having gained some experience in colposcopy, the examiner will
easily be able to position the colposcope
in front of the introitus with one movement so that only minor adjustments with
the focusing handle are necessary to at-
tain a sharp image. A colpophotograph
can then be taken immediately.
Here it becomes evident how important it
is that the colposcope be mounted on a
solid swivel arm or mobile tripod. At a
working distance of 24 cm (or better yet,
30 cm) any additional manipulation using
a swab-holding forceps or a long
anatomic pincette can be managed and
biopsies can be taken under colposcopic
view.

2.2.2 Cervical Smear

The Papanicolaou smear is taken by
swirling a cotton swab over the external
cervical os prior to the application of
acetic acid. If the colposcopic findings are
suspicious, an additional smear can be
taken under observation. The green filter
with which all colposcopes are equipped
should be inserted for a more detailed
view of the vasculature. Photographing
through this filter is not recommended,
however, because the pictures tend to be
underexposed and lacking in detail. This
problem can be overcome by opening the
lens to a wider aperture, but doing so
delays the examination.

2.2.3 Schiller's Test

Schiller's test is used to localize atypical
epithelial areas. A cotton swab dipped in
Lugol's iodine solution or normal iodine
tincture is used to paint the cervix. I use
iodine tincture because it stains the
epithelium more intensely. The epithelium normally stains dark brown,
owing to its high glycogen content. Atypical or inflamed epithelium has a low
glycogen content and stains only slightly
or not at all.
Schiller's test is rather unspecific, and I
do not use it in every case. Schiller originally suggested it be used for macroscopic
differentiation of cervial findings. Consequently, it should be implemented when
the colposcopic findings are unclear, but
most of all before a biopsy is taken or
when another diagnostic procedure such
as conization is planned.
Only with the help of Schiller's test is it
possible to clearly differentiate between
normal and abnormal or atypical
epithelium. Other supportive tests exist,
but I do not use any of them. For example,
toluidine blue solution is reported to allow
for better differentiation between atypical

and normal epithelium. I have only limited experience with its application in the vulval area.

Negatol has, so far as I am concerned, little value as a diagnostic aid. The solution requires a considerable dilution, or it causes cauterization and scab formation. For therapeutic use, negatol is nonetheless a very good drug.

2.3 Colpophotographic Documentation

Early practitioners of colposcopy could demonstrate their observations only by recording them in the form of diagrams. These drawings were always produced after completion of the examination and were often difficult to interpret. A good colpophotograph, on the other hand, provides much stronger proof of the examiner's observations. Despite the undoubted value of hand-drawn diagrams for didactic purposes during training and postgraduate teaching, colpophotography is a far superior method of documentation in clinical use.

Even today, colpophotography is considered extremely difficult; the general opinion is that only a few experts are capable of taking really good pictures. I believe this is no longer true. As already mentioned, I have been working with a stereo camera for 21 years. It takes two 18 × 24 mm stereopictures that are adequately sharp to be enlarged to any required size for documentation and projection. After processing, the stereo slides can be assessed with the help of a specially designed stereo viewer (Fig. 2.8).

Recording and storage of slides, however, poses something of a problem in providing ready access to a patient's slides. Several possibilities have been developed. First, slides can be filed in special vinyl jackets and placed in the patient's records. Alternatively, the slides in their special jackets can be stored in a special filing index. A third possibility is to keep the slides in a special cabinet – a method proven over many years. I use the slide cabinet manufactured by Abodia of Bre-

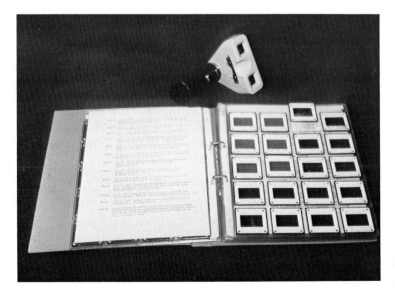

Fig. 2.8. Stereo slide series with special viewer for continuing education purposes.

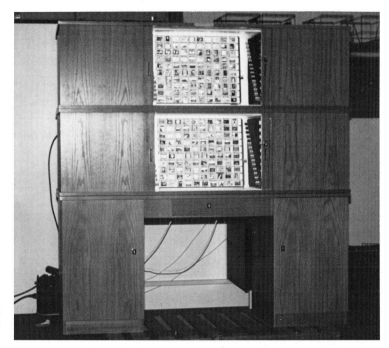

Fig. 2.9. Slide cabinet with an addition; total capacity is 6000 slides.

men. It stores up to 3000 slides on mobile metal frames with 100 slides per frame. On the back wall of the cabinet there is a backlit frosted glass pane similar to those used for viewing x-rays. In the bottom of the cabinet are shelves and drawers for storing folders and other equipment (Fig. 2.9). This cabinet can be expanded at any time by stacking a second cabinet on top of the first. Abodia also makes smaller slide cabinets.

Colleagues who want to acquaint themselves with colposcopy may begin with an autodidactic course that will familiarize them with the most commonly occurring colposcopic situations. For this purpose I have put together several color stereo slide series for viewing with a special viewer that requires no maintenance. It does not have its own light source, so it must be held against an artificial or natural light source for viewing. A battery-operated viewer is also available (Fig. 2.8).

The picture quality is excellent. I often use such slide series in giving courses in colposcopy, and they can be purchased on request. Over the years I have continually improved the slide series: The introductory course now includes 180 color slides and the advanced 200 color stereo slides. Forty sets of each series allow 40 persons to participate in each course, the courses taking 6 hours. The use of video transmission has already been mentioned.

I believe that colpophotographic documentation offers a definite advantage in detecting and documenting changes of the uterine cervix as well as the vagina and vulva. When comparing prints of one patient taken at different times, it is frequently possible to identify more colposcopic detail than seen at the actual examination. This type of repetitive documentation is also particularly valuable for the exchange of information among colposcopists.

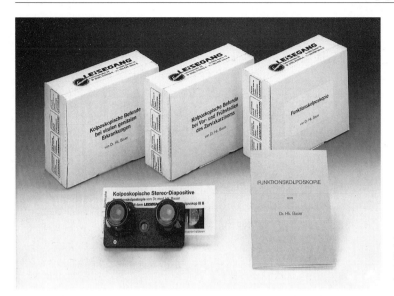

Fig. 2.10. Color stereo slide series for continuing education courses with the stereo viewer.

Colposcopic slides present a wonderful opportunity for postgraduate training because the presence of the patient is no longer required. As long ago as 1955, GLATTHAAR noted: "Colpophotography – like routine chest x-rays – will make a quantitative and qualitative analysis of colposcopic findings not only feasible but it will also render an invaluable contribution in the field of medical education!" Stereophotography of living cervical epithelium allows interesting observations to be made. Epithelial growth and vascular changes can be documented over short or long periods. Valuable knowledge of the epithelial type and its expansion is gained, because in comparison with two-dimensional photographs, three-dimensional presentation permits better recognition of such fine details as irregularity of the surface contour. Colpophotographs allow the diagnoses of less experienced examiners to be verified and confirmed by senior colleagues, closing the informational gap created by the somewhat personal and subjective nature of earlier colposcopic assessments.

Important comparative conclusions can be drawn when colpophotographs are viewed together with the cytologic smear and the corresponding histologic section. Keeping this option in mind, the choice between hand-drawn diagrams and colpophotographic documentation obviously favors the latter, since drawings cannot achieve the same conclusive proof as photographs. We all know the difficult beginning that colposcopy had when compared to cytology with its sound documentation. I therefore consider stereocolpophotography as a definite diagnostic improvement. Every colposcopist should be able to perform it with no loss of time and no major expense. A further advantage is that the slides can be used to produce good color prints to serve as a record in the patient's file.

At the Second Workshop of the study association Cervix Uteri, now the Association for the Study of Cervical Pathology and Colposcopy, important aspects involving colposcopic documentation were the topic of a roundtable discussion. It was agreed that although stereo slides are without doubt a suitable method of documentation for routine use by the private practitioner, prints are required in hospitals and polyclinics. Despite the considerable technical progress that has been made, Polaroid prints do not equal the quality of slides, not to mention their substantially higher cost. Prints of excellent quality can be made from slides at any time and in whatever size is required. The only disadvantage of slides is the time involved in processing.

The significance of colposcopic documentation was also stressed at the third World Congress for Cervical Pathology and Colposcopy. It is to be hoped progress will continue to be made in this direction, forcing the examining physician at some point to keep records of all colposcopic findings. Color photographic documentation lends itself perfectly to this purpose. I have already mentioned an additional method of documenting colposcopic findings. The use of a video camera attached to the colposcope plus a monitor for viewing has proved to be very satisfactory, and further technical progress is being made in this area. For example, the pictures viewed on the monitor can now be photographed. Our goal is to ensure continued technical advances in the documentation of colposcopic findings.

Finally, I would like to quote HANS HINSELMANN, who wrote in a letter to his student MENKEN in 1952:

> "The fact that epithelial changes of the cervix can now be recorded with such precision opens a new dimension for colposcopy..."

My introduction of colposcopy was the first step in what is for mankind the so very significant exploration of the genital mucosa. That my students were able to take the second step fills me with an immense satisfaction.

3: Classification and Explanation of Colposcopic Findings

A good nomenclature should be simple, easily understood, and clear, since it forms the basis for communications between colposcopists. Until recently, German colposcopists adhered to the old nomenclature of HINSELMANN. For years there have been attempts to reach an international acceptance of a classification useful to everyone. This problem was thoroughly discussed at the second World Congress of Cervical Pathology and Colposcopy in Graz in 1975.

3.1 Systems of Classification

The committee on colposcopic nomenclature of the Association for the Study of Cervical Pathology and Colposcopy, a section of the German Society for Gynecology and Obstetrics, has also dealt with this problem since 1974. HINSELMANN's terms *Grund* (groundstructure) and *Felderung* have been replaced by *punctation* and *mosaic*. The term *transformation zone* is now used instead of the traditional customary German word Umwandlungszone. The latest colposcopic nomenclature, modified as explained below, is used in this atlas and presented in Table 3.1. Group I, normal findings, does not differ from the international interpretation of terms. In group II, various findings, however, is contrary to international nomenclature, which lists these in group III. I consider it better, for didactic reasons, to present the benign findings in groups I and II and the abnormal or atypical findings in group III. I took the term papilloma/condyloma out of group II and placed it in group III as an "abnormal or atypical finding". We often find histologic atypias evident under papilloma/condyloma. In addition, I moved the term *iodine-negative area* from group II to group III. Other deviations occur within the abnormal (atypical) findings (group III), in particular the term *atypical (abnormal) transformation zone*. Findings that cannot be evaluated make up group IV.

The term *atypical transformation* zone elicits pronounced differences in opinion among authoritative colposcopists, probably because of the extreme difficulty in defining distinct criteria for this condition. During colposcopy we are dealing with an image of living tissue, which is continually changing. It is therefore impossible always to obtain a conformity with the histologic appearance. The colposcopist normally examines the *surface* of the cervix and if possible the endocervix for epithelial and vascular changes. Obviously, changes located below the surface and therefore invisible to the colposcopist cannot be evaluated. The situation is further complicated by the fact that the histopathologist often describes only epithelial changes while connective tissue – or, even more important, blood vessels – are not evaluated. The basis of the atypical (abnormal) transformation zone is the so-called white epithelium, which stains white when 3% acetic acid solution is applied. The atypical transformation zone is discussed in greater detail in Chapter 4.3.4. More indepth explanation for the remaining colposcopic terms and

Table 3.1 Classification of Colposcopic Findings as Used in This Atlas

I. Normal findings
    a. Original squamous epithelium
    b. Original columnar epithelium
    c. Transformation zone

II. Various findings
    a. Polyps, Cysts, and other changes of the cervix, vagina, and vulva
    b. Erosion
    c. Inflammation
    d. Atrophy

III. Abnormal (atypical) findings
    a. Iodine-negative area
    b. Punctation/mosaic (fine to coarse)
    c. Leukoplakia (fine to coarse)
    d. Atypical transformation zone – white epithelium
    e. Papilloma/Condyloma
    f. Findings suggesting carcinoma (ulcer; exophytic or atypical vascularization)

IV. No evaluation of colposcopic findings possible
    (eg Squamocolumnar junction, hemorrhaging, anatomic difficulties)

their interpretation is given later in this text. As already mentioned, the application of 3% acetic acid solution is mandatory.

To repeat: in classifying colposcopic findings into four groups, I considered it best to present a progression in which the normal findings (group I) are given first, followed by various findings (group II) and *then* by the abnormal or atypical findings (group III). In contrast, the international recommendation is to include the abnormal (atypical) findings in group II. Group IV (in which evaluation of the findings is possible) is mentioned specifically in the descriptions of individual colpophotographs in the atlas portion of this book.

Tables 3.2 and 3.3 present the colposcopic criteria for atypical (abnormal) findings based on BUSCH and modified according to my conceptions to enable differentiation and, more important, prognostic classification of findings. As in Papanicolaou's classification for cytology, I consider such a classification very important for early detection of carcinoma in women. A classification scheme can be rubber-stamped or preprinted on every examination form, saving the examiner from writing lengthy descriptions. A definite advantage of the breakdown into groups is that the colposcopist is forced to categorize findings, and lengthy notes are unnecessary.

It is not my intention to diminish the importance of written descriptions of colposcopic findings; they are still significant. In fact, in cytology, written descriptions of findings have recently been preferred.

In Table 3.2, **groups I–II** (unsuspicious findings) include squamous epithelium with a recognizable junction; squamous epithelium/columnar epithelium; also ectopic columnar epithelium, transformation zone, and various findings such as polyps, cysts, and other changes of the cervix, vagina, and vulva such as erosion, inflammation, or atrophy.

Group III a includes those findings that cannot be definitely diagnosed after a single colposcopic examination, for example, in the case of minor bleeding or

Table 3.2 Classification of Colposcopic Findings (modified according to BUSCH)

Group	Colposcopic Findings
I, II	Unsuspicious
IIIa	Difficult evaluation, follow up after a short interval
IIIb	Mild atypical findings, biopsy is not necessary, follow up
IV .	Severe atypical findings, biopsy mandatory
V	Suspicious of carcinoma

severe inflammatory changes. Those findings listed in Table 3.2 as abnormal: unsuspicious, biopsy not necessary are categorized in group IIIb.

Group IV includes highly suspicious findings that require biopsy.

Group V includes findings in which carcinoma may be suspected on macroscopic grounds and colposcopic findings such as severe atypical vascularization and irregular surface contours are also evident.

Although Australian and North American study groups have included punctation, mosaic, and leukoplakia as well as atypical vascularization under the heading atypical (abnormal) transformation zone, I suggest, in line with the international nomenclature, that punctation, mosaic, and leukoplakia be dealt with as separate groups.

I consider it very important that colposcopic findings be described exactly as they are observed without the interjection of histologic terminology. Fortunately, the combined term "leukoplakia/parakeratosis" has been dropped. This was a case of a colposcopic term being linked with a histologic term, although we all know that histologically leukoplakia is not always identical with parakeratosis.

The role of vascularization has been particularly studied by the research group of STAFL and KOLSTAD. I would like to point out that these authors worked with a significantly higher magnification than the 10× to 15× magnification generally

used in routine practice. This lower power is normally sufficient for evaluation, but is does not permit us to make the same fine differentiation of atypical vascularization as STAFL and KOLSTAD do. For everyday examinations a physician need only recognize the presence of atypical vessels; their individual form is of only academic value. It cannot be stressed enough that the entire colposcopic picture must be evaluated, with especially remarkable abnormal changes being recorded by the examiner.

For example, if mosaic and punctation are found on the edge of a transformation zone, these are naturally classified as abnormal findings. In this case the examiner must decide whether the abnormal changes necessitate a biopsy. The criteria presented in Table 3.3 can help: considerably altered surface level, marked white staining of the epithelium, and so on.

3.2 Explanation of Colposcopic Terms

3.2.1 Original Squamous Epithelium

Original squamous epithelium consists of normal squamous epithelium located distal to the last gland opening. This occurs in about 5% of sexually mature women. The percentage increases markedly in women during menopause. (More details are given in section 4.1.1.)

Table 3.3 Colposcopic Criteria for Atypical (Abnormal) Findings

	Unsuspicious: No biopsy necessary	Suspicious: Biopsy mandatory
Mosaic	Regular Fine – unaltered surface level Acetic acid reaction +	Irregular Altered surface level Acetic acid reaction ++
Punctation	Regular Fine – unaltered surface level Acetic acid reaction +	Irregular Altered surface level Acetic acid reaction ++
Leukoplakia	Fine, slightly raised	Scaly, papillomatous surface level Vulnerability
White epithelium	Fine – level even or slightly raised Acetic acid reaction +	Acetic acid reaction ++ Persistent alteration of surface level Vulnerability
Vascularization	None or normal inter- capillary interval Normal	Atypical: bizarre, broken off, cork- screwlike comma-shaped intercapillary interval Normal
Epithelial defects	Erosion	Ulcerated, exophytic

3.2.2 Columnar Epithelium

Ectopic columnar epithelium on the cervical surface is common and is usually physiologic. Initially one can identify merely a red spot, and only after application of 3% acetic acid will the fine or coarser grapelike structures of the columnar epithelium become apparent. In the presence of inflammation a more or less pronounced vascularization is added. (More details are given in section 4.1.2.)

3.2.3 Transformation Zone

This condition is most frequently seen in women during their reproductive years, and it can appear in a variety of combination forms. The squamous epithelium may predominate, with only a few ectopic islands being seen. Alternatively, the major portion of the cervix may be covered by columnar epithelium, and squamous epithelium will be found only at the edges, where it grows over the ectopy or forms islands by metaplasia. Within transformation zones of longer standing, so-called

gland openings are visible. They may be closed or open. They are characterized by a vascular network that resembles tree branches. Larger closed glands are called Naboth's cysts (mucous cysts). (For further details see section 4.1.3.)

3.2.4 Polyps, Cysts, and Other Changes

First of all, several types of **polyps** can develop in the ectocervix, the endocervix, or the uterine cavity. Their surface may be covered to a greater or lesser degree by metaplastic squamous epithelium or solely by columnar epithelium. Combinations of both are most common. The origin of the polyps cannot be determined colposcopically; this requires histologic examination.

Vaginal cysts may be congenital abnormalities or may develop subsequent to trauma. The congenital form often represents a cyst of the Gartner duct or, in those encountered in the upper third of the vagina, a remnant of müllerian epithelium will sometimes be identified.

The remaining cysts usually occur after delivery or plastic surgery.

A rare condition is the **endometriotic cyst,** which appears through the colposcope as a collection of small blood-filled vesicles.

Almost as rare is **adenosis** located in the area of the posterior fornix. It is characterized by the development of columnar epithelium or transformation zone in this region. Histologically, it has probably developed from the müllerian duct. The cases I have observed so far all had the typical transformation zone seen at the cervix. (See section 4.2 for details.)

A special variety of benign cervical polyp formation is the so-called **polypoid transformation zone,** which occurs during pregnancy or in women taking oral contraceptives. The tissue proliferation can be so massive that it requires surgical removal like an ordinary polyp of the cervix. During pregnancy, decidual polyps must also be taken into consideration in the differential diagnosis. (See section 4.2.2 for details.)

3.2.5 Erosion

True erosion is characterized by a localized epithelial defect. The exposed stromal tissue can be recognized by its more or less pronounced vascularization. In many instances one cannot ascertain whether erosion conceals dysplasia, carcinoma in situ, or even frank carcinoma. If no healing is achieved by local treatment (within about 4 weeks), histologic examination is mandatory. (See section 4.2.8 for details.)

3.2.6 Inflammation

Severe infection increases the difficulty of evaluating the colposcopic image, just as it does the cytologic evaluation (Papanicolaou smear). Diffuse vascular engorgement due to inflammatory reaction does not allow any detail to be identified, and the assessment is frequently hampered by small hemorrhages. Such findings must be considered suspicious so long as complete healing is not achieved by local therapy. (Punctation-like vascularization is explained in section 4.2.9.)

3.2.7 Atrophic Changes

Epithelial atrophy is characterized by a thin, transparent epithelium. It is most commonly encountered in postmenopausal women, but it also occurs in younger patients with ovarian insufficiency subsequent to premature ovariectomy and in primary sterility. Beneath the thin epithelium one can often identify vessels that tend to bleed easily. Such diffuse or local hemorrhages may appear in large numbers. (See section 4.2.10.)

3.2.8 Atypical (Abnormal) Colposcopic Findings

Undoubtably, the principal ongoing problem is to classify all visible conditions systematically. In endeavoring to do this, I am fully aware that individual findings in certain cases might be classified differently. For the newcomer to colposcopy, however, I consider it best to adhere to a schematic evaluation.

My own approach to any classification was always guided by the colposcopic appearance rather than the histologic interpretation, knowing that these need not correspond. We now know that colposcopic findings at the epithelial level, involving fine alterations (for example, fine slightly white epithelium or fine punctation/fine mosaic) are harmless, although technically called abnormal. Histopathologic classification, unfortunately, does not provide for these slight changes. The result is a major discrepancy between colposcopic and histologic findings, but this does not constitute a disadvantage of colposcopy. The reverse situation, in which colposcopically benign-appearing lesions proved atypical histologically, could be disastrous for the patient. I have observed such minor abnormal changes for 25 years, and to date I have never observed the development of a severe histologic atypia.

3.2.9 Iodine-negative Area

Generally, the so-called iodine-negative test is less important to colposcopy than the 3% acetic acid test. This does not mean we should spurn Schiller's test if questionable findings are involved. We know that, apart from colposcopically abnormal epithelium, there are a number of benign iodine-negative alterations. This is particularly true for inflammatory epithelial changes and likewise for columnar ectopy. That is why Schiller's test is less significant than the application of 3% acetic acid solution. The method is valuable in doubtful colposcopic findings, mostly for differentiating epithelial atypia prior to conization. (See section 4.3.1.)

3.2.10 Punctation

According to WESPI, punctation is characterized by numerous red dots corresponding to the tips of stromal papillae with their capillary loops. Like all the other atypical changes, punctation as a rule is sharply delineated from normal epithelium. Of the two types, fine punctation is usually harmless, whereas coarse punctation must always be considered suspicious, necessitating biopsy for histologic assessment. Coarse punctation was previously termed papillary ground structure.

If punctation extends into the cervical canal, colposcopic assessment becomes rather difficult, and such cases certainly need to be evaluated histologically. (See section 4.3.2.)

3.2.11 Mosaic

The condition known as mosaic impresses by its numerous small tissue fields within a sharply demarcated area. GANSE explains the development of these fields by a boulder-like proliferation of atypical epithelium whereby a mosaic pattern is created because of small epithelial bridges between the individual blocks. Mosaic appears in different forms of tetragonal, rhombic, or bizarre shapes. As with punctation, fine mosaic occurring within the cervical surface is usually harmless. If, on the other hand, this atypia is combined with an elevation and irregularity of the surface contour, the lesion has to be regarded as highly suspicious. (See section 4.3.3.)

3.2.12 Leukoplakia

As with punctation and mosaic, we differentiate between fine and coarse leukoplakia – a distinction that can be clearly recognized even before the application of 3% acetic acid. Under colposcopic visualization, fine leukoplakia presents as a white patch that is usually well delineated from the normal epithelium. The histologic section usually shows a benign hyper- or parakeratosis. Coarse leukoplakia with marked elevation above the epithelial surface requires histologic assessment because of its suspicious nature. (See section 4.3.4.)

Mosaic, punctation, and leukoplakia often appear concurrently. The same principle applies as for individual presentation: The suspicion of malignancy increases when the lesion display elevated or irregular surface contours. A histologic evaluation is then mandatory.

3.2.13 Atypical Transformation Zone

The atypical transformation zone presents a diagnostic problem even for the experienced examiner. The incidence of this finding at colposcopic examination is reported by different authors to be from 0.2 to 3%. Evaluation is based on the criteria for atypical or abnormal colposcopic findings (see Table 3.2). The lesion is usually characterized by an increased vascularity. Vascular atypias may be swollen with a turbid yellowish discolorization. Glandular openings are frequently visible; they appear like punched-out holes, having a reddish base and a circular arrangement of capillaries around the apertures. The openings are either elevated in a papillary fashion or recessed. Irregularities in the surface contour are a particularly suspicious omen.

The atypical transformation zone may include one or more atypical findings, that is, punctation, mosaic, or leukoplakia. Diagnostic determination, however, is the whitness of the epithelium: The more intensely the epithelium stains white and the longer the white stain lasts, the greater the probability of malignancy. The surface contour – that is, the variation in surface level – is also important. These changes generally occur within a transformation zone, and the transitions are smooth. I therefore base my classification on the findings that are most prevalent. The presence of prevailing white epithelium with gland openings and erosive patches, interspersed by only minimal areas of mosaic and punctation, identifies the lesion as atypical transformation zone. Conversely, if areas of mosaic and punctation are dominant, I use these terms to describe the observation. The more atypical the additional findings, the greater is the suspicion of malignancy. Even if the Papanicolaou smear is nega-tive, histologic evaluation is indicated. Of the 0.2 to 3% of cases in which colposcopic findings are abnormal, some authors state that malignant processes can be histologically determined in one third. I consider this outdated. More often we find preliminary stages such as dysplasia and carcinoma in situ – CIN I. (See section 4.3.5.)

3.2.14 Papilloma/condyloma

In general, there are hardly any colposcopic differences between papillomas and condylomas. Histologic assessment shows, in addition to numerous benign changes, a number of atypical changes beginning with slight dysplasia (CIN I) through carcinoma in situ – CIN III. Papillomatous tumors, particularly if they are vulnerable and show severe atypical vascularization, may already be carcinomatous. One should therefore always pay special attention to such changes. (See section 4.3.6.)

3.2.15 Findings Suspicious of Carcinoma (atypical vascularization; exophytic changes; ulcers)

Early cervical carcinoma – microcarcinoma (group 1a) and cervical carcinoma (group 2b) – is distinguished colposcopically by the striking irregularity of the epithelial surface, vulnerability, and atypical vascularization. Amid the areas of coarse mosaic and punctation, one can observe numerous broken-off vessels, so-called corkscrew capillaries, hairpin capillaries, and, especially, vessels of bizarre shape and varying thickness. The assessment of the intercapillary distance is an important aspect, but an ordinary colposcope with a 10× to 15× magnification may not permit detailed evaluation of the capillary network. Another criterion to look for is the so-called adaptive vascular hypertrophy. In all cases of blood vessel alterations the interposition of the green filter proves to be very useful.

The more the carcinomatous growth has advanced, the less detail is visible through the colposcope, because the weakness and bleeding tendency of the tissue interferes with making the observation. For this reason, the diagnosis of advanced carcinoma is easier by direct visualization. (See also section 4.3.7.)

4: The Use of Colpophotographs in Colposcopic Diagnosis

The following color colpophotographs of normal, various, and atypical findings are arranged to present the most important and most frequently occurring colposcopic findings in such a way that they can easily be remembered by newcomers to the method.

GANSE, BAADER, and others take their pictures without a colposcope, using a special camera with bellows and extension tubes (a technically rather costly and time-consuming method). My photographs, explained in the foregoing discussions, are taken through the colposcope during the gynecologic examination. Thus all illustrations were obtained in daily practice in a specialist's consulting office. They represent a cross section of the patients encountered in the daily practice and therefore cannot be claimed comprehensive.

The prints are reproduced without any retouching so that they appear identical to what is seen through the colposcope. Formerly, enlargements were made from the 18×24 mm half-Leica format. For technical reasons, the edges had to be cropped from the 10×15 cm prints, reducing the format to 7.5×9 cm. For this edition, the photos of the new figures were reproduced directly from the half-Leica format, ie, from the slide to 7.5×9 cm prints.

A certain systematic approach is necessary, although this can certainly invite criticism. As already outlined, the classification is always based on the observation as seen through the colposcope. This presents no difficulty regarding the normal colposcopic findings, but problems do arise with the various and atypical findings. Every experienced colposcopist knows, and I must stress this again, that in the latter the colposcopic and histologic findings do not always match. Other authors proceed with their classification primarily from the histologic evaluation and offer three interpretations: negative, suspicious, and positive. In my opinion this approach overemphasizes the detection of carcinomatous lesions. Since we are able to diagnose a benign condition in 90% of all cases with a colposcope alone, I regard the classification presented here as more adequate. This classification is, after all, for the most part in conformity with the suggested nomenclature of the World Congresses of Graz 1975 and Orlando 1978.

Because there is no clear, absolute distinction between "various" and "atypical" colposcopic findings, interpretation is particularly complex. For example, it can be rather difficult to give a colposcopic opinion in the presence of inflammatory changes. A smear from an infected cervix can present a similar problem to the cytologist.

In my opinion, the beginning colposcopist should first become acquainted with the most frequently encountered conditions, which are absolutely benign findings: original squamous epithelium, ectopy, and transformation zone. After achieving sufficient skill in diagnosing the benign cases, one can turn to the more difficult "various findings" (group II) and "atypical or abnormal findings" (group III). Regarding the latter, the atypical transformation zone represents a complex area which can be most difficult to assess.

4.1 Normal Colposcopic Findings

4.1.1 Original Squamous Epithelium

The vagina and cervix are covered by a nonkeratinized squamous epithelium without glands. When examined histologically, the lowest portion at the stromal border consists of a layer of basal cells followed by a layer of parabasal cells. The next cell type is represented by intermediate cells. The surface, which has a honeycomb appearance, is composed of superficial cells with scanty pyknotic nuclei. Hormonal influences on the vaginal and cervical epithelium can be assessed through the colposcope. Patients who are pregnant or take oral contraceptives, frequently demonstrate a livid bluish epithelial tint. Young women with ovarian dysfunction often present with the finding of original squamous epithelium.

During the reproductive years the normal squamous epithelium has a smooth pink surface. Vessels are usually not visible because the epithelium is thick. With advancing age it becomes progressively thinner, allowing the subepithelial vascular network to shimmer through. In Schiller's test, the normal squamous epithelium always stains mahogany brown because of its glycogen content. Where the epithelium is thin, patches with whitish dots may occur, this being referred to as papillary relief surface.

Although the squamocolumnar juncture is usually clearly visible during fertile life, it tends to extend into the endocervical canal in the aging female. A definite assessment about the presence of atypical epithelium can be made only if this juncture is visible in its entirety. In such cases the cytologic (Papanicolaou) smear of the cervix need not be taken.

In young women the incidence of original squamous epithelium covering the whole cervix is at most about 5%.

In such cases it is not possible to disprove the presence of atypical epithelium colposcopically, and a cervical (Papanicolaou) smear is essential. However, epithelial atypia inside the endocervix occurs in only 5 to 15% of fertile women. A completely healed transformation zone does not always permit differentiation of secondary or metaplastic squamous epithelium from the original. In this case, one should take particular care to look for discrete, extremely isolated open glands. According to GLATTHAAR, it is at the juncture of the two epithelial structures with their entirely different biological characters that continuous cervical changes take place. From this, two practical conclusions can be drawn:

1. If colposcopic inspection reveals only original squamous epithelium with no visible squamocolumnar juncture, a conclusive evaluation is not possible and one has to rely on the cytologic (Papanicolaou) smear.

2. The finding of original squamous epithelium in fertile women of childbearing age is usually a sign of ovarian disturbance, – for example – primary sterility.

As already mentioned, we find the squamocolumnar juncture shifting upward into the cervical canal with advancing age. This explains the high percentage of colposcopically detected squamous and atrophic epithelium in older women, especially those who are postmenopausal. Here, the same principle applies as for original squamous epithelium during the reproductive years: Colposcopy alone cannot give a reliable assessment about a premalignant or malignant condition of the uterine cervix. Not infrequently, evaluation of the cytologic smear will also present a diagnostic problem, firstly because cervical changes related to aging may make it difficult to obtain a representative endocervical specimen and, second, because differential diagnosis of a cytologic slide in cases of atrophy is often fraught with difficulty.

Fig. 4.1: Squamous epithelium of the cervix

Patient: 20-year-old nullipara. The external os of the cervix has a horizontal shape and is slightly open. The mucous secretion is transparent and contains small air bubbles.

The border between the squamous and columnar epithelium can be seen at the anterior and posterior cervical lips. A so-called "gland opening" is visible at about 4 o'clock, indicating secondary metaplastic growth of the squamous epithelium.

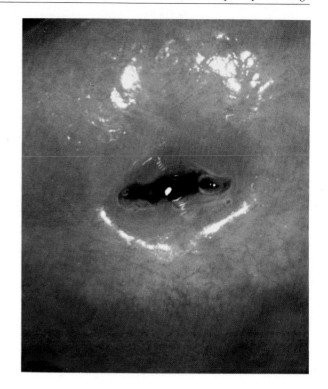

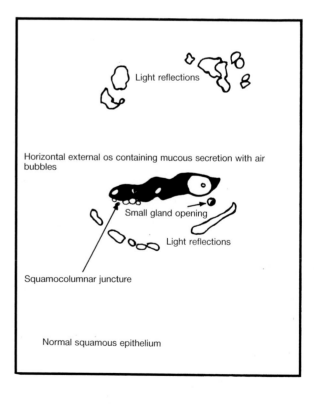

Fig. 4.2: Original squamous epithelium of the cervix

Patient: 33-year-old nullipara with primary sterility. The external cervical os is slightly gaping, exhibiting clear mucous secretion. The squamocolumnar epithelial juncture is not visible, so the occurrence of atypia cannot be established colposcopically. The finding of original squamous epithelium is a sign of inner secretory disturbances. An absence of inflammation can be stated with certainty.

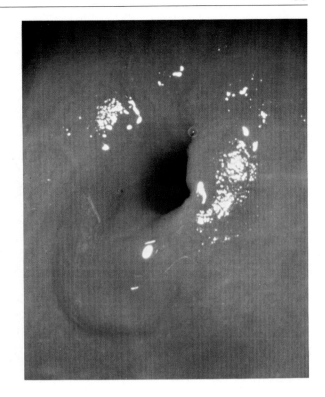

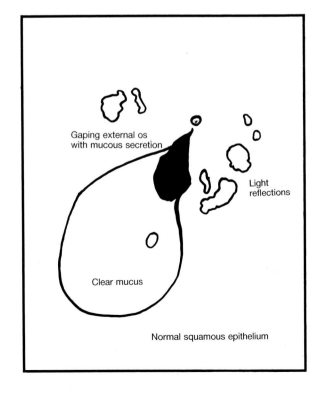

Fig. 4.3: Original squamous epithelium of the cervix

Patient: 36-year-old nullipara. A small amount of mucous secretion is visible covering the external, umbilicated os. The normal squamous epithelium appears pink. In places, small capillaries can be identified through the epithelium indicating slight atrophy.

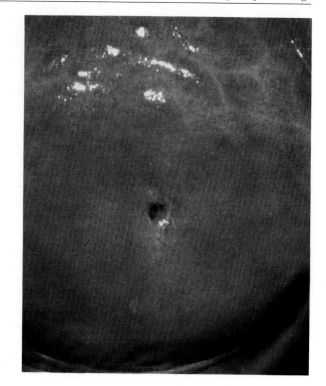

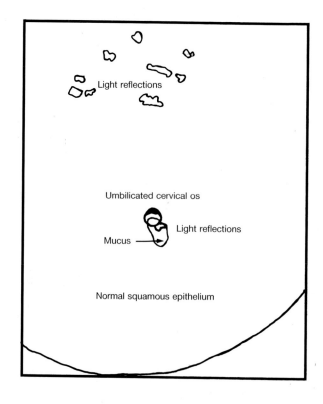

Fig. 4.4: **Original squamous epithelium of the cervix**

Patient: 21-year-old nullipara. The external cervical os is open, with clear mucous secretion. The squamocolumnar epithelial juncture is just barely visible through the opening, the cervix has a pale pink appearance, and there are numerous light reflections.

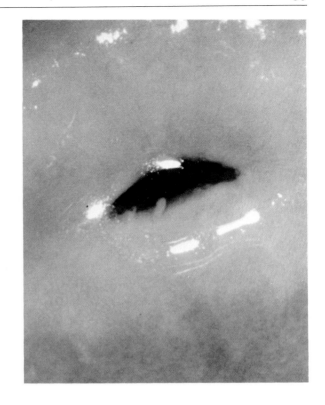

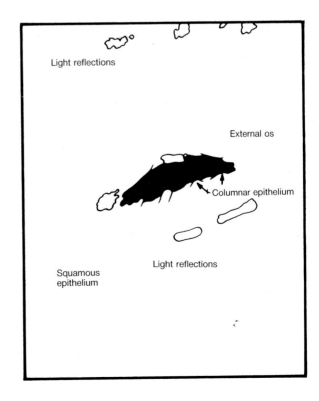

Fig. 4.5: Original squamous epithelium of the cervix (See also Fig. 4.6)

The cervix of a 52-year-old para 1 with regular menstruation. No squamocolumnar epithelial juncture can be seen in this view. It is first visible upon spreading the external os.

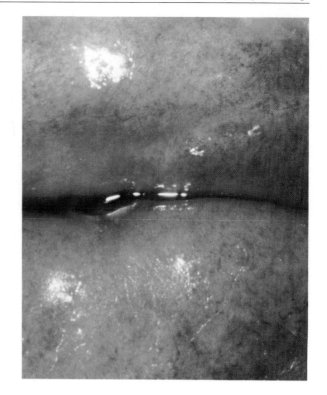

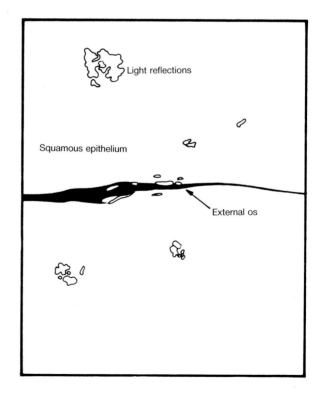

Fig. 4.6: Original squamous epithelium of the cervix – transformation zone

Same patient as in Fig. 4.5: Upon spreading the external os the squamocolumnar epithelial juncture is clearly visible, and colposcopic evaluation is now possible. Clearly recognizable, especially around the external cervical os, are an unsuspicious transformation zone, mucous secretion in the cervical canal, and a small polyp.

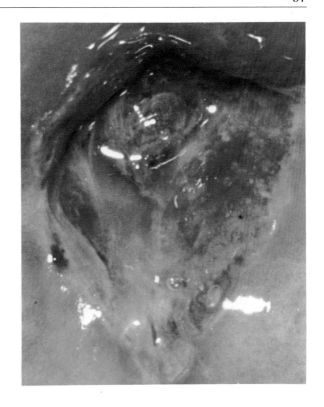

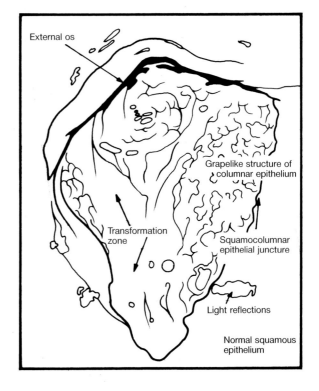

4.1.2 Ectopic Columnar Epithelium

The appearance of columnar epithelium on the cervical surface is a common finding which is, in most cases, quite physiological. Ectopy develops by means of an external shift of the endocervical mucosa in toto, ie, ectropionization. This ectropion consists not only of superficial columnar epithelium but also of glands and loose subepithelial stromal tissue.

The special significance of the 3% acetic acid test can be convincingly demonstrated in this frequently encountered condition. Prior to acetic acid application only a red spot (erythroplakia) is visible. Afterwards, the columnar epithelium takes on the appearance of a fine or coarse grapelike structure. The white, grapelike appearance of the columnar epithelium is probably caused by swelling or protein precipitation. After the 3% acetic acid solution has been applied, one must wait, sometimes as long as 30 seconds before the grapelike pattern can be best visualized. This effect often disappears just as quickly.

Gynecologists who do not perform colposcopic examinations usually refer to these areas as pseudoerosion or erosion. In this age of colposcopy, the terms "pseudoerosion" and "erythroplakia" should be discarded, while "erosion" should be used only to describe true erosion.

Ectopy can sometimes be identified in newborn or prepubertal females. Not infrequently, such findings remain unchanged for a long time. During the reproductive years the squamocolumnar juncture is located at the ectocervix in most women and as such is easily visible through the colposcope. In these patients it is possible to exclude a premalignant or malignant process of the cervix with an accuracy of almost 100% by colposcopy alone. With advancing age the squamocolumnar juncture moves into the endocervical canal, which means that colposcopic evaluation in older women becomes doubtful. Often ectopy is accompanied by vaginal discharge and inflammation, which can be more pronounced if the ectopic columnar epithelium covers a large surface area. Under these circumstances it may be difficult to give a colposcopic opinion. Inflammatory changes within the area of ectopy may also be secondary to cervicitis. Such cases, of course, require local treatment (a detailed management is beyond the scope of this atlas).

The columnar epithelium of the cervix produces an alkaline mucus. Exposure to the acid vaginal environment is likely to be responsible for an increased secretion with secondary inflammatory reaction. During pregnancy and also after administration of oral contraceptives, the area of ectopy can demonstrate edematous and polypoid changes.

These findings are occasionally difficult to interpret because of the pronounced vascularization. Colposcopic and cytologic reevaluation at shorter intervals is indicated.

Fig. 4.7: Ectopic columnar epithelium

Patient: 26-year-old nullipara. The fine grapelike structure of the columnar epithelium is clearly visible only after application of 3% acetic acid. The resulting protein precipitation and coagulation removes mucous secretions, allowing easy inspection of the entire border between squamous and columnar epithelium. Lateral to this juncture are nabothian cysts and some gland openings. Such a finding in the absence of any symptoms is completely normal and, when as unequivocal as in this patient, justify excluding any suspicion of malignancy on the basis of colposcopy alone.

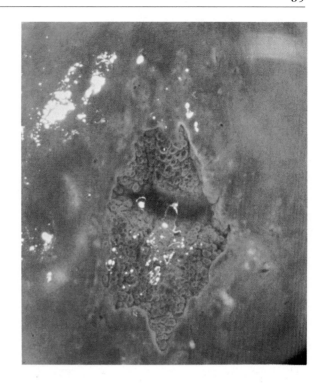

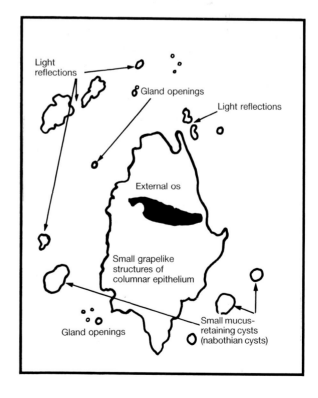

Fig. 4.8: Ectopic columnar epithelium

Patient: 16-year-old nullipara. Narrow ectopy of columnar epithelium; the border with the normal squamous epithelium of the cervix is visible in its entire length. The finding is physiologic and absolutely benign. The patient has no symptoms and therefore requires no treatment.

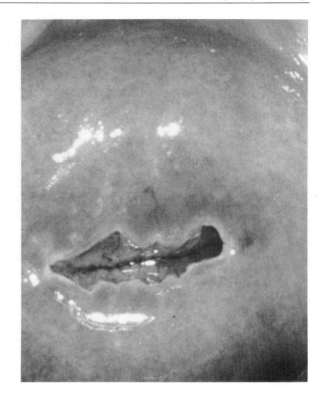

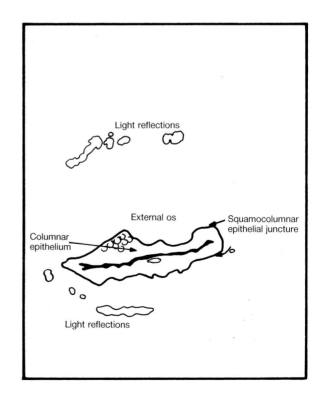

Fig. 4.9: Ectopic columnar epithelium; extensive cervical laceration (Emmet laceration)

Patient: 25-year-old 8 weeks after forceps delivery. A large tissue defect is seen near the posterior external cervical os. The coarse grapelike structure of the columnar epithelium is clearly visible. The external os gapes wide open.

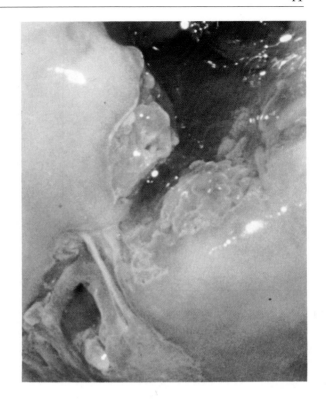

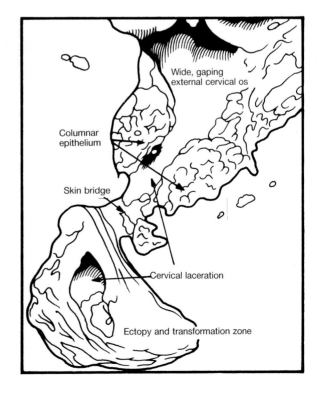

Fig. 4.10: Ectopic columnar epithelium

Patient: 18-year-old nullipara. The slightly oblique cleft of this external os disproves the general textbook opinion that nulliparas have a round, umbilicated cervical opening. The use of 3% acetic acid renders the fine grapelike structures of the columnar epithelium clearly visible, and the border to the squamous epithelium can be identified in its entirety. Again, we are dealing with an absolutely benign and physiologic condition.

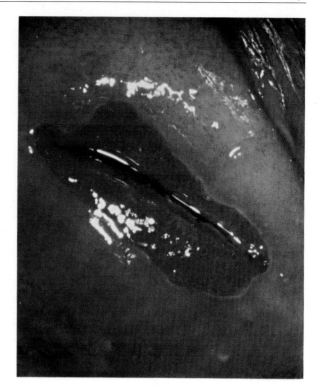

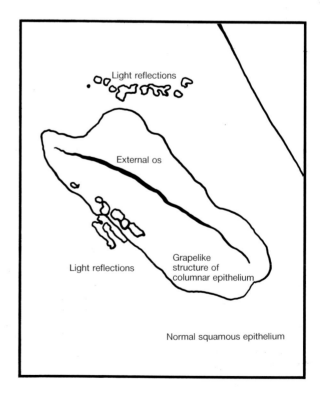

Fig. 4.11: Polypoid, bluish ectopic epithelium following use of oral contraceptives

Patient: 30 years old. The squamous epithelium and also part of the columnar epithelium have a distinctly bluish livid tint that indicates either pregnancy or use of oral contraceptives. Such considerable proliferative changes are seen less frequently in recent years because the estrogen and gestogen content of oral contraceptives has been reduced. This 30-year-old patient had taken oral contraceptives with predominantly gestogenic content. Sometimes the tumorlike appearance may confuse even the colposcopist. An additional finding is the presence of a few yellowish nabothian cysts caused by mucus retention.

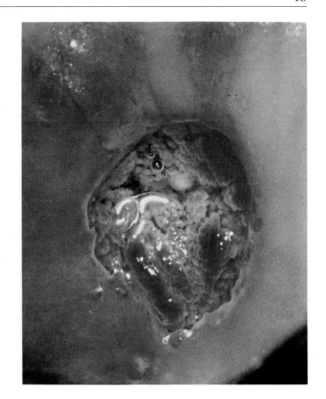

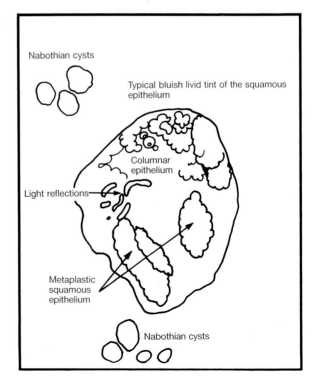

Nabothian cysts

Typical bluish livid tint of the squamous epithelium

Columnar epithelium

Light reflections

Metaplastic squamous epithelium

Nabothian cysts

Fig. 4.12: Polypoid, bluish ectopy

Patient: 25-year-old primigravida. The coarse grapelike structures of the columnar epithelium are edematous and show some degree of bluish livid coloration. The neighboring squamous epithelium has the same color tone. Such proliferative changes occur, as demonstrated in Fig. 4.11, in women who are pregnant or take oral contraceptives. In this case a pregnancy was confirmed.

This kind of finding is sometimes difficult to differentiate from decidual polyps (See also Figs. 4.32 and 4.33).

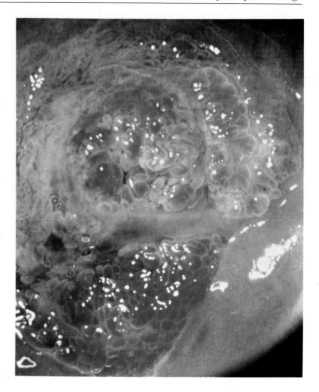

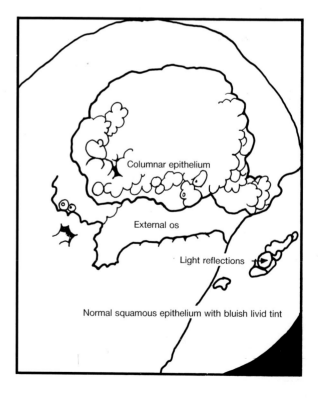

Fig. 4.13: Ectopic columnar epithelium; transformation zone on the periphery

Patient: 49-year-old nullipara. This patient presented with a history of severe hormonal dysfunction coupled with recurring secondary amenorrhea leading to longterm therapy with estrogens and gestogens. The positive response to the hormone therapy can be seen in the unsuspicious nature of the ectopy and the transformation zone in the surrounding area.

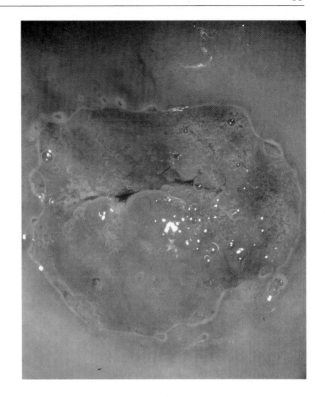

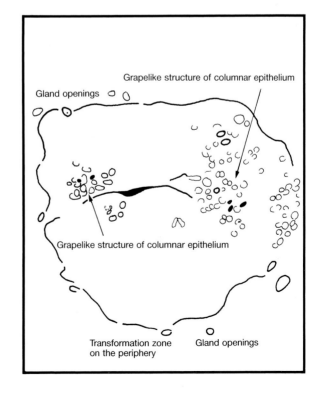

4.1.3 Transformation Zone

The transformation is the most common colposcopic finding in women during their reproductive years. The histologic term for transformation zone is *meta-plasia,* and it simply means that colum-nar epithelium is replaced by squamous epithelium. Numerous combinations are possible. The squamous epithelium may dominate the cervical surface, with ec-topic columnar epithelium being iden-tified only in the form of small islands. In contrast, most of the cervix may be cov-ered by ectocopy, with small areas of squamous epithelium developing by means of metaplasia originating below the columnar ectopy or from its peripher-al borders. Older transformation zones exhibit so-called gland orifices, which may be closed or open.

The colposcopic observation may thus indicate the presence of opposing colum-nar and squamous epithelium. The bor-der between the two linings, which ap-pears to shift continually, was previously referred to as the "battle zone." Topo-graphically, this juncture is of great sig-nificance because when malignant cervi-cal changes occur, they do so at this site in over 90% of cases.

The replacement of columnar epithelium by squamous epithelium at the transfor-mation zone is thought to take place in two ways. According to HAMPERL, squa-mous epithelium originating in the periphery progressively invades the co-lumnar epithelium, continually replacing it. The second mode (FISCHER-WASELS) consists of indirect metaplasia: Squamous epithelium develops *within* the area of ectocopy from undifferentiated cells originating beneath the columnar epi-thelium.

The developing metaplastic squamous epithelium can cause retention of mucus, leading to the formation of nabothian cysts. The retained mucus is often con-centrated and thickened while the cover-ing epithelium has a whitish, glossy ap-pearance; branching vessels are often visible running across the cyst wall.

The so-called "gland openings" most probably develop in response to in-creased mucus pressure by forming a channel between the covering metaplastic squamous epithelium and the buried cer-vical crypts of columnar ectopy. The se-cretion through the aperture is often clear-ly visible during colposcopy. As described in the previous chapter, the same state-ment applies to the transformation zone as to ectopy: If the border of a normal transformation zone in a fertile female allows full inspection, the diagnosis of a benign condition can be assumed with almost 100% certainty.

Fig. 4.14: Transformation zone

Patient: 33-year-old gravida 2. An area of ectopy with transformation zone is present mainly at the anterior cervical lip. As repeatedly emphasized, this process of regeneration of the cervical epithelium is commonly seen in women during their reproductive years. Tongues of squamous metaplasia grow from the outer edges in the direction of the cervical os, here and there surrounding islands of columnar epithelium. A number of nabothian cysts – small, yellowish, transparent – can be identified. The external os contains mucus with air bubbles.

This patient has had an intrauterine contraceptive device in place for two years, the threads being visible in the right lower corner of the colpophotograph.

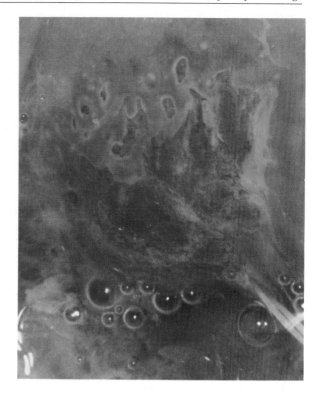

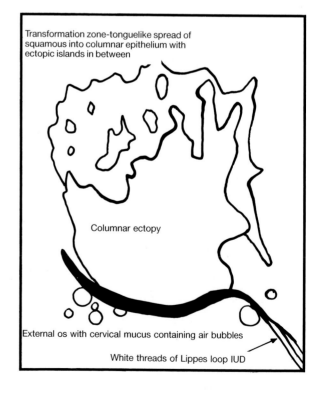

Transformation zone-tonguelike spread of squamous into columnar epithelium with ectopic islands in between

Columnar ectopy

External os with cervical mucus containing air bubbles

White threads of Lippes loop IUD

Fig. 4.15: Transformation zone

Patient: 44-year-old para 3. An ectopy with transformation zone is present mainly at the anterior cervical lip; the transformation zone has progressed farther at the posterior cervical lip. Ectopic islands are visible between 4 and 6 o'clock. The external os contains several large air bubbles. In addition, mucus is evident at the posterior cervical os. The transformation zone is relatively fresh.

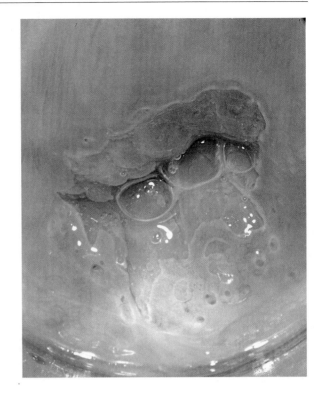

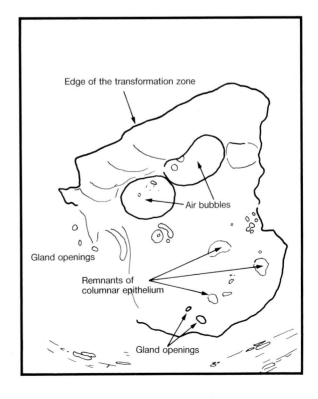

Edge of the transformation zone

Air bubbles

Gland openings

Remnants of columnar epithelium

Gland openings

Fig. 4.16: Transformation zone (See also Fig. 4.17)

Patient: 30-year-old para 2. An ectopy and transformation zone is present mostly at the posterior cervical lip, also exhibiting a nabothian cyst (mucus retention cyst) somewhat below the surface. A proliferative tendency of the columnar and the squamous epithelium is clearly evident and is related to use of oral contraceptives. Moreover, there is distinct whitish squamous epithelium on the left side of the colpophotograph which became visible after application of 3% acetic acid. This patient has had two normal deliveries.

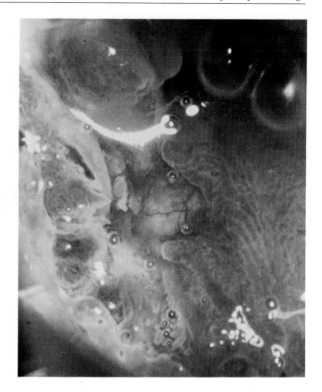

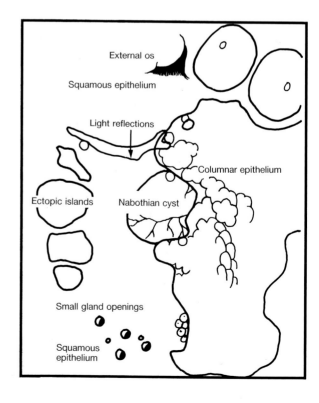

Fig. 4.17: Transformation zone (See also Fig. 4.16)

Patient: same as in Fig. 4.16. Eight years later, the patient presents with a distinct shift in the squamocolumnar epithelial juncture toward the cervical canal. This is most evident at the posterior cervical lip. Two polyps covered by squamous epithelium have developed in the cervical canal. After application of acetic acid, white epithelium is seen within the transformation zone at the anterior cervical lip. Secondary finding: several air bubbles.

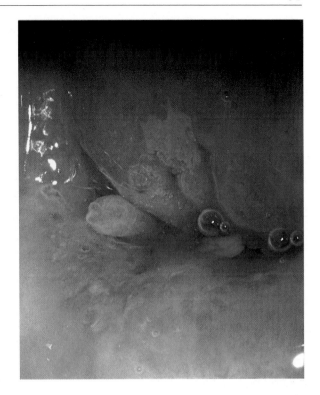

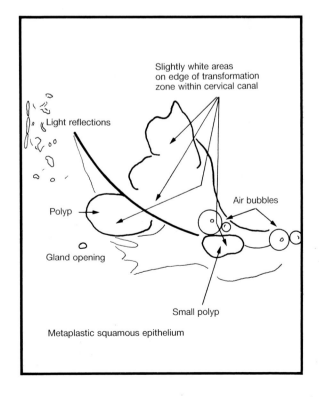

Fig. 4.18: Transformation zone

Patient: 46 years old. The transformation zone is demonstrated, showing large islands of exceptionally noticeable ectopy. The metaplastic squamous epithelium has either grown from the peripheral edges or from deeper down (reserve cells), thereby replacing the columnar epithelium and leaving large circular areas exposed. In addition, gland openings consisting of cervical crypts surrounded by metaplastic squamous epithelium are visible.

The development of squamous metaplasia is typical for women of childbearing age. Only with approaching menopause and its inherent change in hormonal function will this process of epithelial transformation be arrested.

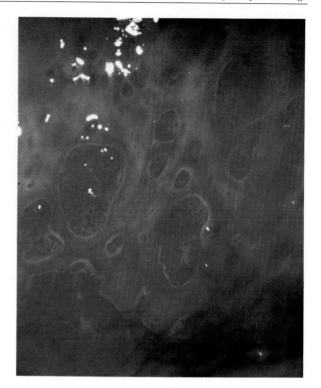

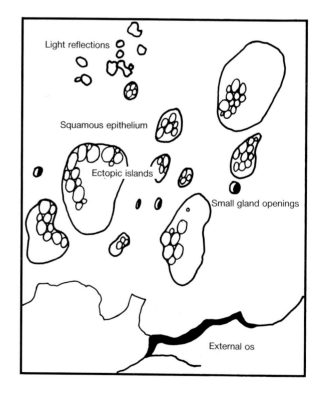

Light reflections

Squamous epithelium

Ectopic islands

Small gland openings

External os

Fig. 4.19: Transformation zone

Patient: 13-year-old with intact hymen. Whitish grapelike structures of the columnar epithelium are visible as well as ectopic islands, particularly at the anterior cervical lip. The columnar ectopy is invaded by tongues of squamous epithelium. This finding in a 13-year-old patient with an intact hymen represents a physiologic condition not requiring any treatment. Hormonal function can also be deduced: The presence of columnar epithelium at the ectocervix signifies normal function.

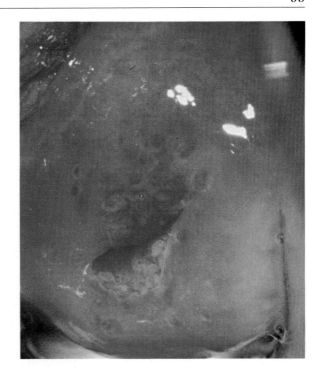

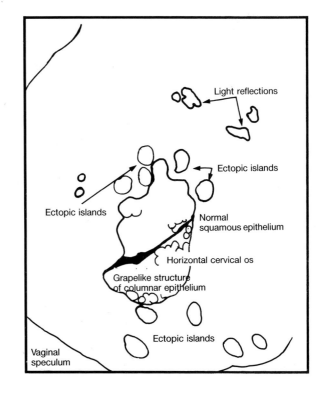

Fig. 4.20: Transformation zone, Copper-T IUD during expulsion

Patient: 25-year-old nullipara. This patient came to the clinic complaining of minimal lower abdominal discomfort. The intrauterine contraceptive device was removed. The transformation zone has a physiologic appearance not requiring any form of treatment.

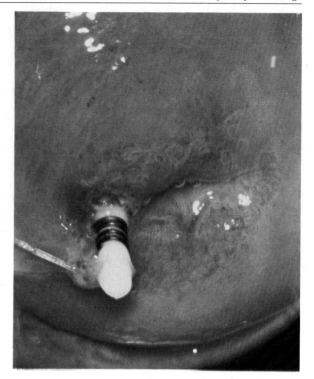

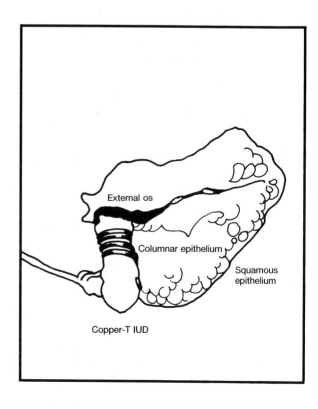

Fig. 4.21: Open transformation zone

Patient: 40 years old. This case illustrates an old, so-called open transformation zone showing a vascularization pattern. The term *open transformation zone* refers to the appearance of numerous gland openings that characterize the colposcopic picture. Their development is explained by squamous metaplasia taking place within the ectopy (differentiation of reserve cells) and from the outer edges. The ectopic columnar epithelium is to a lesser or greater extent replaced, and cervical crypts become surrounded by squamous epithelium. The gland openings can be identified mainly at the posterior cervical lip. The vessels are partly dilated. The slightly gaping external os contains transparent mucus, indicating that this 40-year-old patient is ovulating.

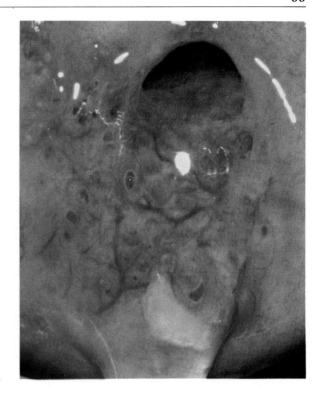

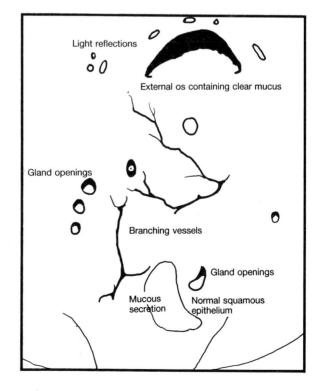

Light reflections

External os containing clear mucus

Gland openings

Branching vessels

Gland openings

Mucous secretion

Normal squamous epithelium

**Fig. 4.22: Old completed
transformation zone
(See also Fig. 4.23)**

Patient: 48 years old. Several
nabothian cysts with pro-
nounced vascularity are present. The posterior cervical lip
shows a somewhat thickened
squamous epithelium as seen
in early keratosis.

This type of transformation
zone exhibiting marked vascularization cannot always be
interpreted easily. Colposcopic
reevalution should be performed at regular intervals
(every 6 months), and a yearly
cytologic smear is advisable.

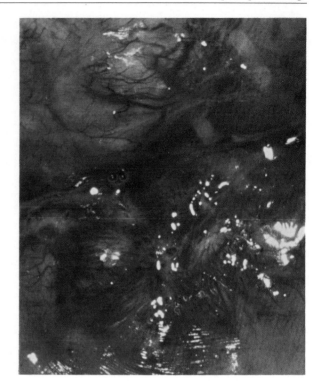

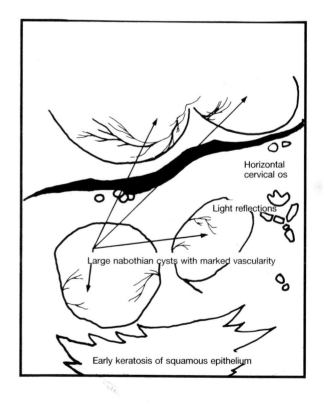

Horizontal
cervical os

Light reflections

Large nabothian cysts with marked vascularity

Early keratosis of squamous epithelium

**Fig. 4.23: Old transformation
zone (See also Fig. 4.22)**

Patient: same as in Fig. 4.22.
The same patient 7 years later
with complete involution of the
severe vascularization seen in
Fig. 4.22. The 55-year-old patient now presents with an
unsuspicious transformation
zone.

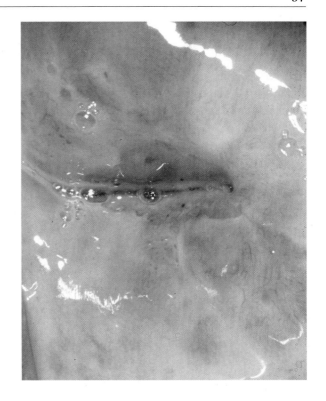

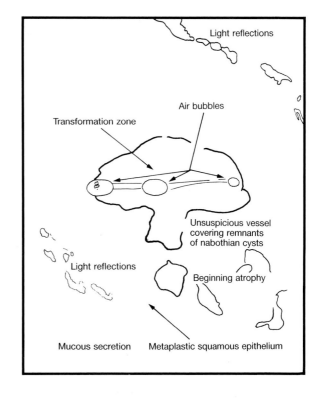

Fig. 4.24: Red area/erythroplakia (See also Fig. 4.25)

Patient: 20-year-old nullipara. This finding is observed when no 3% acetic acid solution is applied. One can merely recognize a red area, mainly around the posterior cervical lip. Macroscopically, this is defined as erythroplakia, a term that does not exist in colposcopic nomenclature. Therefore a differential diagnosis is not possible.

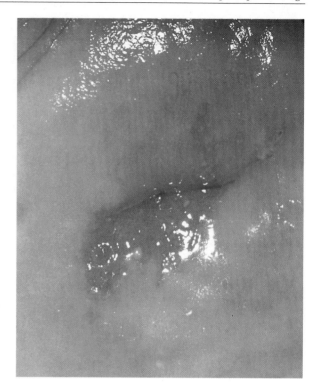

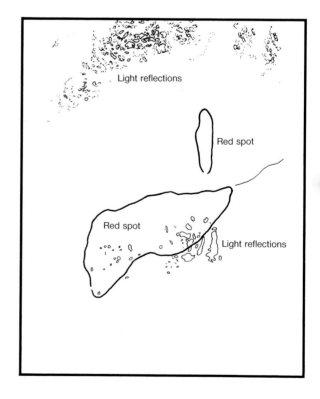

Fig. 4.25: Transformation zone (See also Fig. 4.24)

Patient: same as in Fig. 4.24. The same patient following the application of 3% acetic acid. Here numerous small nabothian cysts are clearly recognized, indicative of an unsuspicious transformation zone.

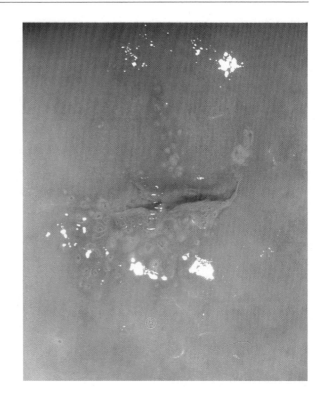

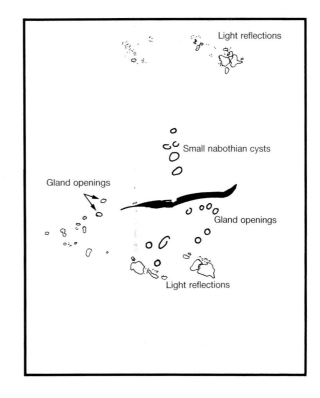

Fig. 4.26: Large polypoid transformation zone (See also Fig. 4.27)

Patient: 28-year-old nullipara. This large polypoid structure is actually a transformation zone that involves the entire cervical os, leaving only a small gap which can still be seen anteriorly. The surface is covered by columnar and metaplastic squamous epithelium.

Such hypertrophic proliferations are often present in women taking oral contraceptives. This 28-year-old nulliparous patient has been using an oral contraceptive for several years. A reduced estrogen and gestogen content in these preparations has made this kind of finding rarer.

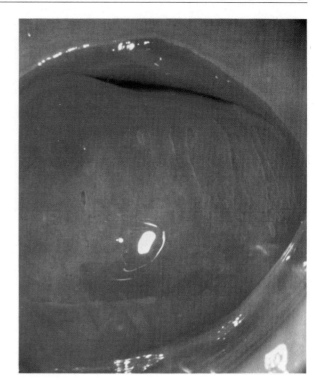

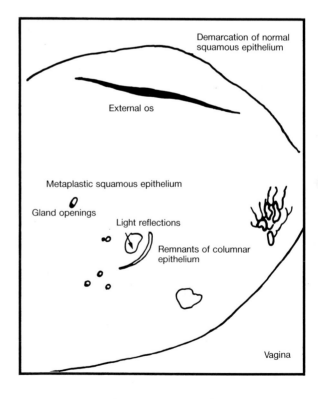

Demarcation of normal squamous epithelium

External os

Metaplastic squamous epithelium

Gland openings

Light reflections

Remnants of columnar epithelium

Vagina

Fig. 4.27: Small transformation zone (See also Fig. 4.26)

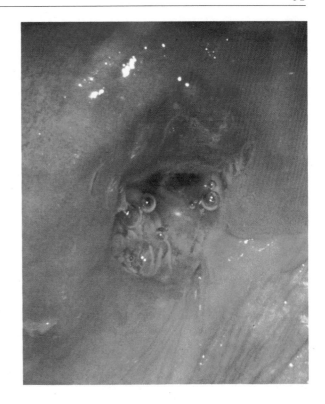

Patient: same as in Fig. 4.26. This colpophotograph was taken half a year later in the same patient as in Fig. 4.26 after removal of the previously large polypoid transformation zone. Oral contraception was also discontinued at the time. When the patient later became pregnant , the cervical hypertrophic proliferation immediately recurred, regressing only after delivery.

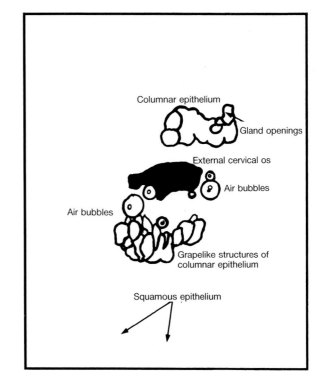

4.2 Various Colposcopic Findings: Polyps, Cysts, and Other Benign Changes

This section deals with colposcopic findings such as polyps, polypoid changes, and several cyst formations of the cervix, vagina, and vulva. Some other benign lesions of the vaginal canal are also described.

4.2.1 Cervical Cysts

A frequent observation in the cervix is the formation of mucus-retaining cysts called nabothian cysts. Their development has already been explained in section 4.1.3. During ectopic replacement, squamous epithelium may grow over columnar epithelium, occluding the mucusproducing crypts with subsequent formation of retention cysts. Rarely, a fibroma or myoma may occur, and colposcopic differentiation is not possible. Another rare finding is endometriosis, appearing in the form of small blood-filled vesicles. Histologic confirmation often cannot be obtained.

4.2.2 Cervical Polyps

Polyps are quite commonly found on the cervical surface and more frequently in the endocervical canal, but also at the urethra. It is not possible to distinguish between a cervical and a protruding uterine polyp by colposcopy; this requires histologic examination. Decidual polyps are observed during pregnancy (See Figs. 4.33 and 4.34).

4.2.3 Vaginal Polyps

Granulation polyps are usually visible after hysterectomy and other vaginal surgery. These lesions tend to bleed easily and may, owing to the inflammatory reaction at the surface, sometimes cause diagnostic difficulties for the inexperienced colposcopist. Biopsy for hystologic evaluation is indicated if the lesion enlarges or fails to disappear after cauterization (e g), with silver nitrate. Special caution must be exercised if polipoid tissue develops at the vaginal vault subsequent to surgical treatment for a premalignant or malignant condition.

4.2.4 Vaginal Cysts

Vaginal cysts do occur. According to LIM-BURG, two thirds of all patients with vaginal cysts have no symptoms. The origin cannot always be determined histologically. These cysts may develop congenitally, deriving from Gartner's (wolffian) ducts or, more rarely, from the epithelium of the müllerian ducts. For the most part, these congenital cysts are uncommon; and when identified, they often are found on the vaginal walls.

Furthermore, vaginal cysts can follow traumatic events. They will be found in the posterior wall or in the lower third of the vagina after perineal lacerations, episiotomies, or vaginal plastic surgery. Vaginal adenosis in conjunction with this condition has been reported in the literature, and I have seen several such cases in recent years (See Fig. 4.38). Opinions vary as to their originating in the vaginal columnar epithelium. The most popular theory is that they develop from the müllerian ducts. Some authors also believe that cysts can develop in response to birth trauma. All the cases I have observed were in nulliparous patients. Colposcopic findings usually show ectopy with transformation zone. These changes are therefore absolutely benign. (At this time, I do not want to go into the problem of stilbesterol in connection with the development of vaginal carcinoma; this is a frequently observed occurrence in the United States.)

4.2.5 Vulval Cysts

Lesions may also be identified at the vulva, an area that has received insufficient attention from colposcopists. Now and then, small cysts are present as a result of inflammatory or traumatic changes. The *Bartholin gland cyst,* of course, can in most instances be identified without magnification. Small *sebaceous cysts* are frequently visible.

Another important indication for vulval colposcopy is the presence of pruritus, and fine erosive areas are often first recognized by colposcopy.

4.2.6 Dystrophy Versus Dysplasia

The new nomenclature regarding vulval changes differentiates between dystrophy and dysplasia. I disagree with this classification because the clinical term *dystrophy* is used interchangeably with the histologic term *dysplasia.* Despite general agreement atrophic genesis should no longer be considered dystrophy, in my experience this is not correct. In postmenopausal older women especially, outright atrophic changes are often seen in the cervix as well as the vagina and vulva. The estrogen deficiency observed in such cases can be reversed with proper treatment.

More recent research supports my view: Dystrophy seems to have a mixed genesis; that is, both atrophia and hyperplasia are seen. Vulval changes that were formerly called *Kraurosis vulvae* are also called *Lichen sclerosus et atrophicans.* They are characterized by marked epidermal atrophy which may be the basis for the development of leukoplakia by secondary epithelial hyperplasia (Grimmer). These lesions can give rise to carcinomatous precursors and to cancer.

Such coarse forms of leukoplakia are also observed in younger women of childbearing age. Histologically this usually involves carcinoma in situ (CIN III) or Morbus Bowen (See Fig. 4.53).

The modern term *dysplasia,* a histologic designation, corresponds to the histologic changes CIN I to III (that is, mild, moderate, or severe dysplasia) carcinoma in situ. A clear differentiation between benign changes (dystrophy) and precancerous changes (dysplasia) is not possible, in my opinion, because of the smooth transition between the two. Melanoma must be taken into consideration if bluish nodules are found near the vulva. This particularly malignant epidermic cancer is fortunately rarely seen at the vulva (See Figs. 4.56 and 4.57).

4.2.7 Sexually Transmitted Lesions

Cases of *herpes genitalis* have increased greatly in recent years. *Condylomas* are also frequently observed. Further, the occurrence of numerous inflammatory processes in the vulval area need to be mentioned (it is not possible to go into detail in this atlas).

It follows from all that has been stated that: *The examiner should inspect the vulva at every gynecologic examination!*

Fig. 4.28: Large nabothian cyst

Patient: 53 years old. A large nabothian cyst is present at the anterior cervical lip, partly covering the external os. Cysts of this dimension are relatively rare. They are usually multilocular and contain a yellowish mucus. The branching vessels have a completely regular pattern and must be regarded as absolutely benign.

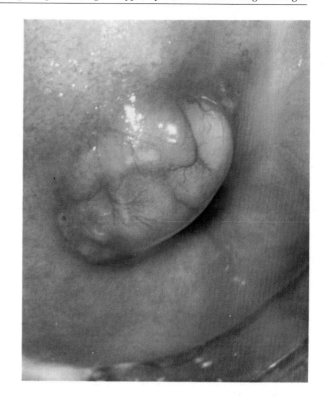

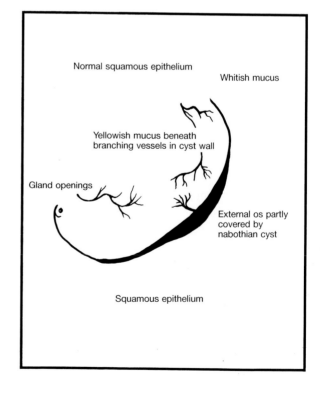

Normal squamous epithelium

Whitish mucus

Yellowish mucus beneath branching vessels in cyst wall

Gland openings

External os partly covered by nabothian cyst

Squamous epithelium

Fig. 4.29: Large cervical polyp

Patient: 49-year-old nullipara. The larger part of this polyp is covered by inflamed metaplastic squamous epithelium; some columnar epithelial remnants can still be identified. The anterior cervical lip illustrates an area of fine mosaic, whereas leukoplakia is faintly visible posteriorly. This 49-year-old nulliparous patient has had two previous cervical polypectomies with benign histologic findings.

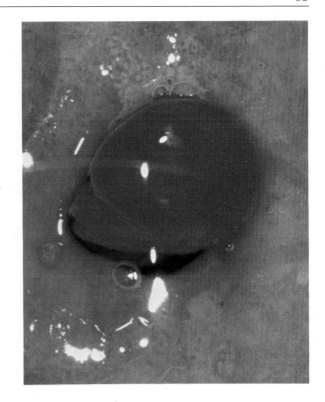

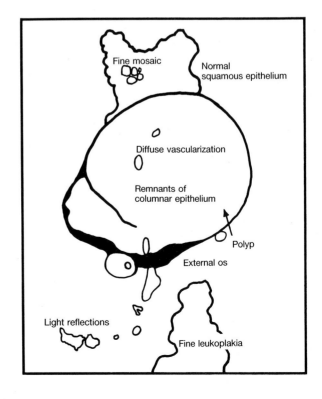

Fig. 4.30: Large endocervical polyps

Patient: 45-year-old multipara. The surface of the polyp is inflamed and hemorrhagic. It is definitely a tumorous structure. Such large polyps are usually located in the uterine body. To determine the type of polyp requires histologic clarification. In this case, histologic assessment showed the 45-year-old multipara to have a uterine polyp.

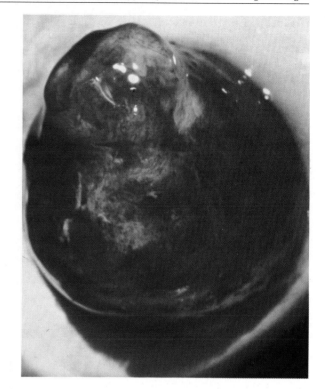

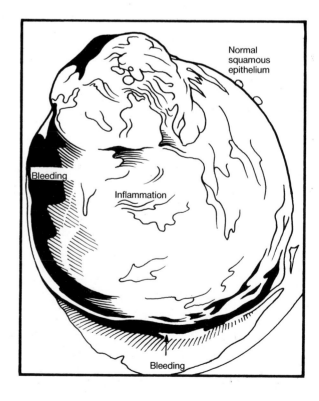

Fig. 4.31: Large uterine polyp

Patient: 45 years old. This polyp, occupying the external os, has led to a dilatation of the cervical canal. Colposcopically it is, of course, not possible to differentiate between an endocervical and a uterine polyp. The surface here is covered partly with columnar and partly with metaplastic squamous epithelium.

The histologic examination revealed a polyp of uterine origin. This 45-year-old patient suffered from recurrent severe menorrhagia. Uterine polyps had already been removed on two previous occasions by dilatation and curettage. Vaginal hysterectomy was performed.

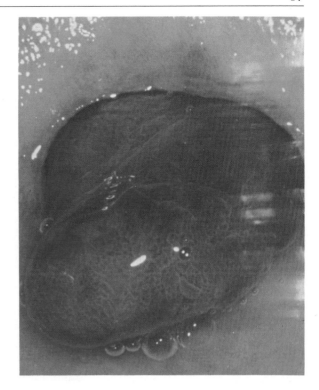

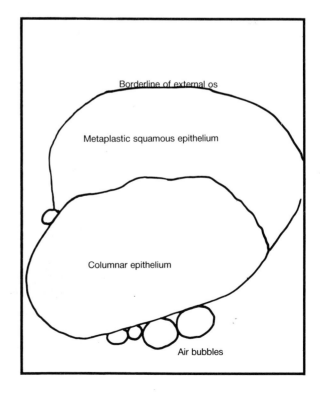

Fig. 4.32: Granulation polyp

Bleeding granulation tissue is present at the vaginal vault following total hysterectomy. When seen through the colposcope it looked like a polyp. On the right side of the picture, squamous epithelium appears to grow over the inflamed granulomatous excrescences.
Such a finding might cause difficulty in the differential diagnosis for the inexperienced colposcopist. Generally, this type of polypoid granulation tissue disappears soon after cauterization (e g, with silver nitrate).

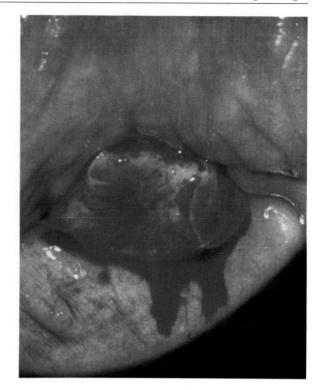

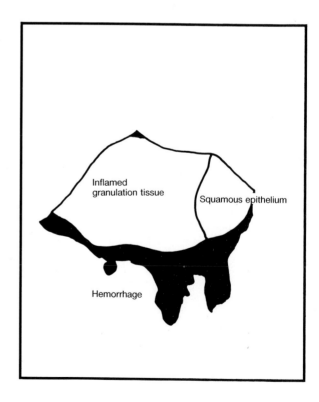

Inflamed granulation tissue

Squamous epithelium

Hemorrhage

Fig. 4.33: Decidual polyp

Patient: 33-year-old gravida 2. A slightly hemorrhagic polypoid structure with marked mucous secrection is observed in the cervical canal. Details can be clearly recognized. Such a finding often makes a differential diagnosis difficult (see also the text to Fig. 4.34 for further explanations).

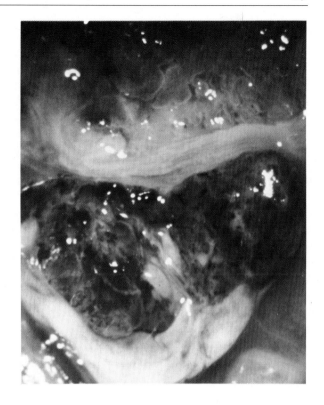

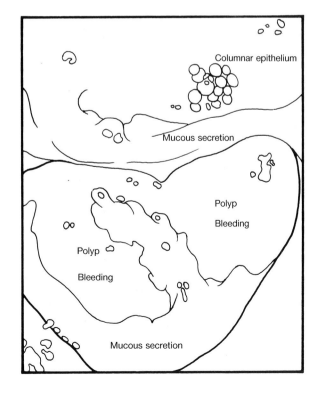

Fig. 4.34: Decidual polyp

Patient: 23-year-old gravida 2. A tumorous atypical transformation zone completely occupies the endocervical canal. Remnants of columnar ectopy can be identified adjacent to squamous epithelium, which turns whitish after application of acetic acid. Furthermore, several atypical vessels are present. Colposcopic interpretation of this lesion is difficult. Even if the cytologic (Papanicolaou) smear in such a case is negative, there is no other choice but to take a directed biopsy of the tumor. Histologic examination of the punch biopsy specimen revealed a heterotopic decidua formation with severe inflammatory reaction, situated within a cervical ectopy.

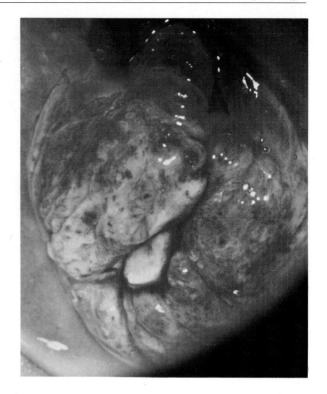

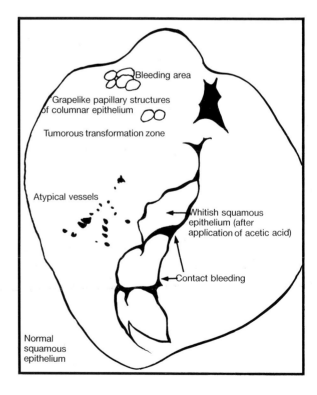

Bleeding area

Grapelike papillary structures of columnar epithelium

Tumorous transformation zone

Atypical vessels

Whitish squamous epithelium (after application of acetic acid)

Contact bleeding

Normal squamous epithelium

Fig. 4.35: Vaginal endo-
metriosis

Patient: 29-year-old para 2. A bluish nodule is visible at the tip of a clinically palpable barshaped nodule. Somewhat lower, the vaginal epithelium shows a bluish discoloration. The patient presented with abdominal bleeding and a dragging pain.

Histologic findings: vaginal endometriosis.

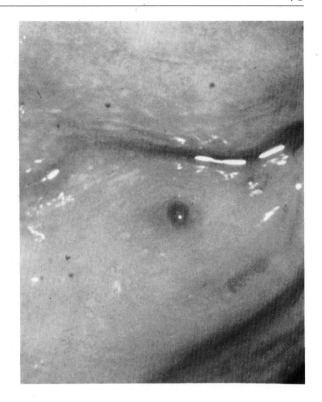

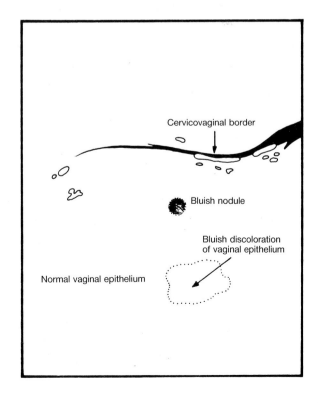

Cervicovaginal border

Bluish nodule

Bluish discoloration
of vaginal epithelium

Normal vaginal epithelium

Fig. 4.36: Vaginal cyst

Patient: 54-year-old para 3. This large cyst has probably developed as a result of trauma during delivery. The patient had no symptoms. The lesion has existed now for 15 years showing no changes. If opened it would possibly drain mucus and old clotted blood.

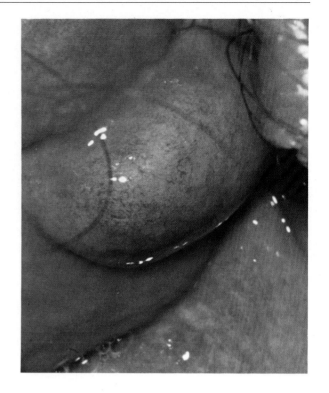

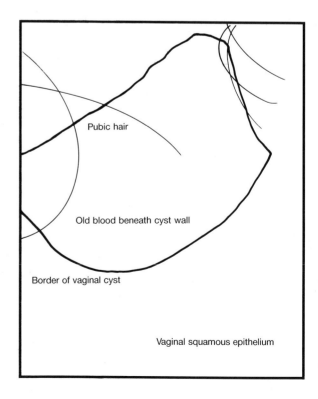

Pubic hair

Old blood beneath cyst wall

Border of vaginal cyst

Vaginal squamous epithelium

Fig. 4.37: Congenital cyst in the lateral vaginal wall, close to the uterine cervix

Patient: 25 years old. The origin of congenital cysts cannot always be determined by histology. In this case the cyst developed from the Gartner (wolffian) duct system. The patient had no symptoms whatsoever, and the abnormality was a purely coincidental finding.

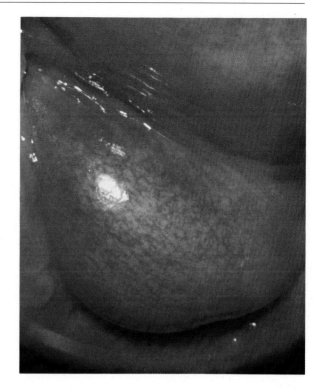

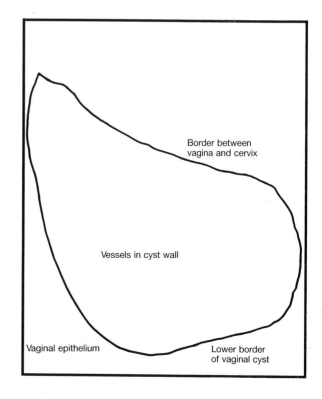

Fig. 4.38: Vaginal adenosis

Patient: 40-year-old nullipara. Columnar epithelium, metaplastic squamous epithelium, and marked vascularization are visible immediately beyond the cervical os at the posterior vaginal wall.

Histologic findings: ectopy with squamous epithelial metaplasia (see 4.1.3).

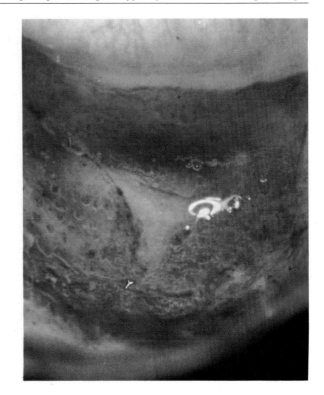

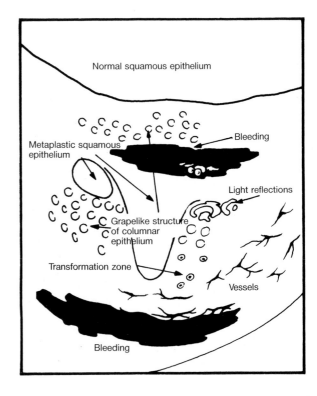

Fig. 4.39: Intact hymen in 8-year-old girl

Injuries at the hymenal ring are more easily assessable through the colposcope than with the unassisted eye. This patient was referred for evaluation of the possibility of rape. The integrity of the hymen could be proved by colpophotographic demonstration.

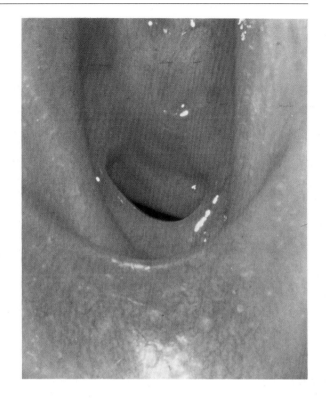

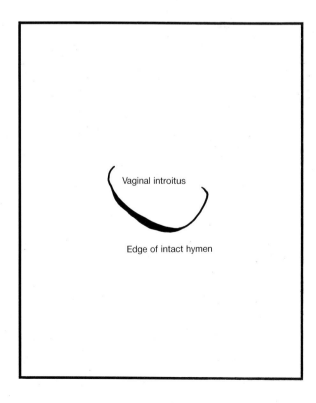

Vaginal introitus

Edge of intact hymen

Fig. 4.40: Large urethral polyp

Patient: 68 years old. This large polyp has a smaller lobe at its proximal portion and is mostly covered by metaplastic squamous epithelium. Furthermore, there are areas of fine mosaic indicating the presence of inflammation.

The 68-year-old patient had reported dysuria and a feeling resembling the sensation found at vaginal prolapse. The lesion was removed.

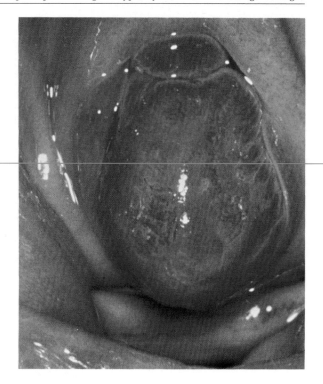

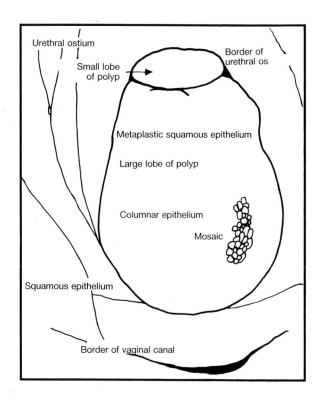

Fig. 4.41: Previous marsupialization of a left-sided Bartholin cyst

Patient: 33 years old. The small aperture of the Bartholin duct at the lower third of the left labium minus can just be identified. A punctation-like reddening of the surrounding epithelium is present.

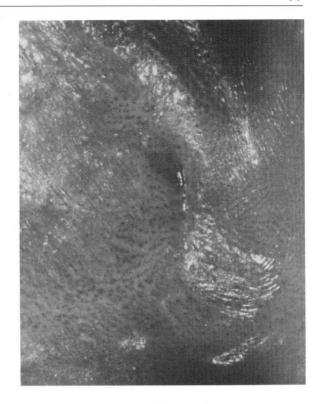

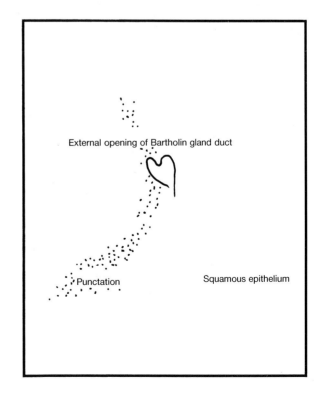

External opening of Bartholin gland duct

Punctation

Squamous epithelium

Fig. 4.42: Vulval erosion

Patient: 24 years old. This rather painful epithelial defect below the vaginal fourchette developed after delivery.
The patient had an uneventful recovery after local therapy.

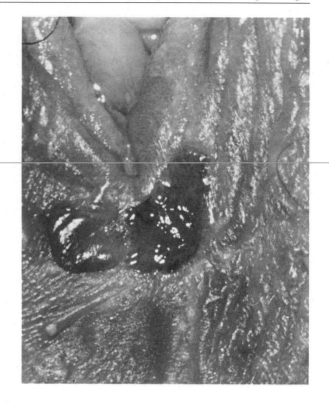

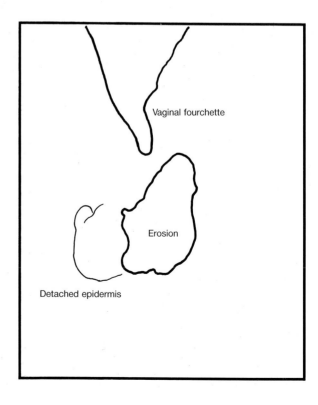

Fig. 4.43: Vaginal cyst

This cherry-sized cyst caused considerable discomfort for the patient. It developed at the vaginal fourchette. Yellowish mucus can be seen inside, and the rather thin wall of the cyst contains completely benign appearing vessels with a treelike branching distribution. It is very likely that this lesion occurred subsequent to an episiotomy.

Histologic findings: unilocular cyst with the inside covered partly by squamous epthelium and to some extent by a single layer of columnar cells.

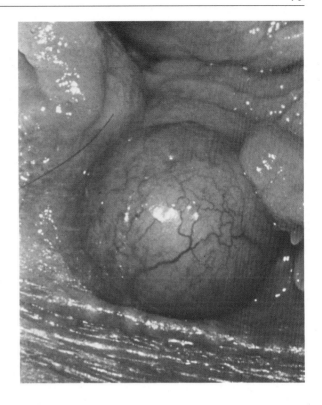

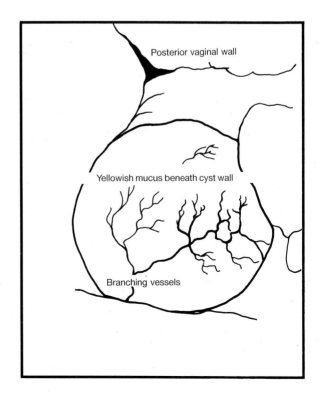

Posterior vaginal wall

Yellowish mucus beneath cyst wall

Branching vessels

Fig. 4.44: Pruritus vulvae (cause: *Pediculus pubis* infestation)

Patient: 19 years old. The patient presented with severe itching elicited by *Pediculus pubis* (crab louse) infestation. Small bluish-gray specks — *taches bleuâtres* or *maculae caeruleae* — are clearly seen on the skin. The nits (ova) are observed fixed to the pubic hair shafts. It is even possible to follow the movement of the lice with the colposcope if they leave the burrow.

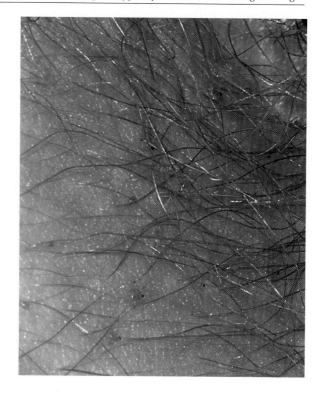

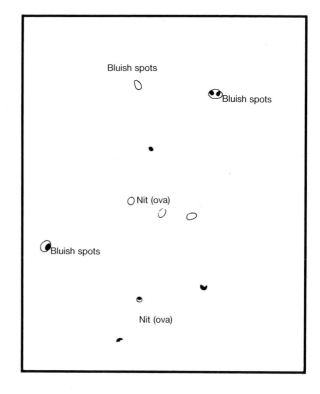

Fig. 4.45: Acute, purulent vulvitis with erosions

Patient: 19 years old. Numerous ulcerations and thick mucoid patches observed near the vulva of the patient led to severe swelling of the entire vulval area. The severe inflammation also caused retention of urine.

Cause: *Candida* mykosis and gonorrhea.

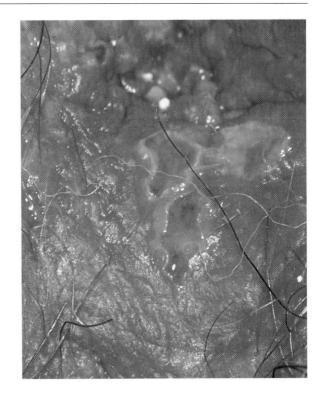

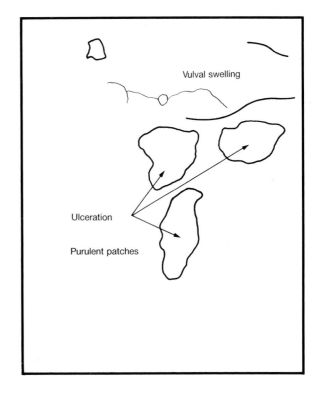

Fig. 4.46: Acute vulvitis with erosions and nodulation

Patient: 42-year-old nullipara. Small ulcerated areas, barely visible with the naked eye, are found at the vulva near the introitus. Small nodules are also present. The patient presented with a severe itching and burning sensation at the vaginal orifice.

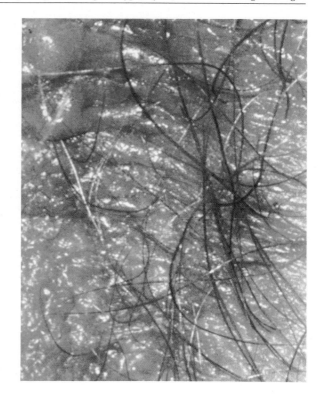

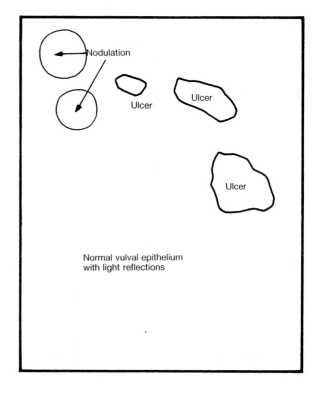

Fig. 4.47: Genital herpes

Patient: 39-year-old para 2. The patient presented with severe pruritus and pustular development at the vulva. Herpes vesicles and erosions are observed.

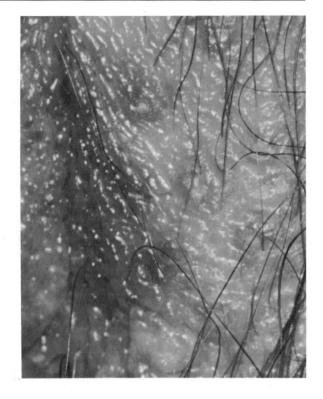

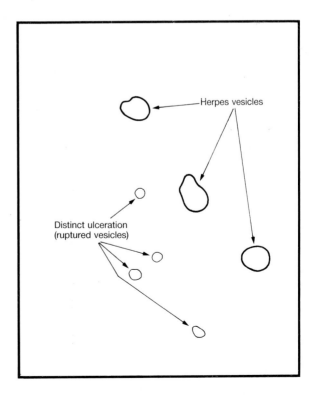

Fig. 4.48: Genital herpes

Patient: 16 years old. The patient presented with severe pruritus. Several herpes vesicles are visible here, some already ruptured and with distinct pit formation.

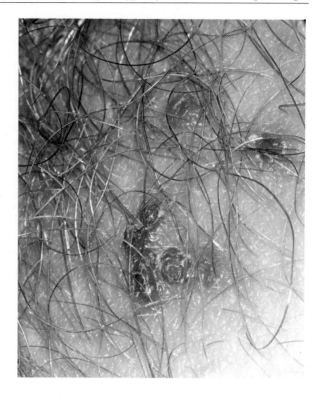

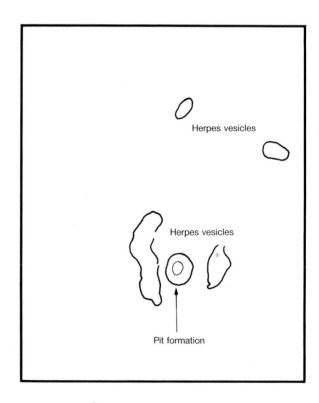

Fig. 4.49: Vulval aphthae

Patient: 30 years old. These whitish plaques surrounded by reddened halos can cause severe pruritus.

The origin is viral, similar to aphthous stomatitis. The lesions healed after the patient received local corticosteroid application.

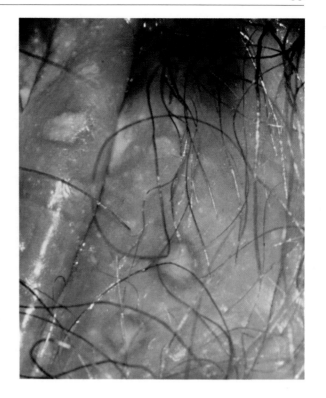

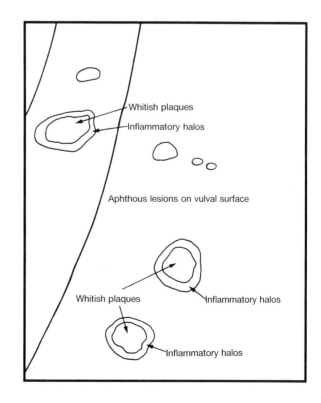

Fig. 4.50: Vulval varices

Patient: 62 years old. A post-menopausal patient with no symptoms.

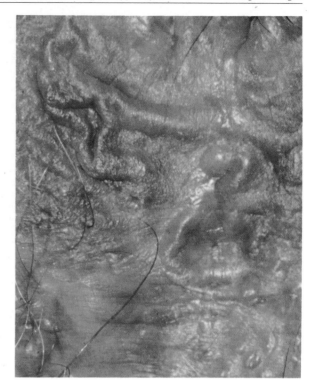

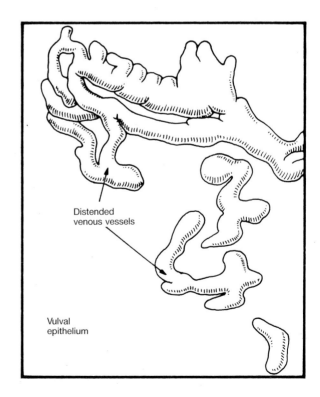

Distended
venous vessels

Vulval
epithelium

Fig. 4.51: Vulval dystrophy

Patient: 60-year-old para 2. The condition now known as vulval dystrophy was formerly called kraurosis vulvae. The term lichen sclerosus et atrophicus is also used. In this case the vulval lips are completely atrophied. The patient had taken estrogen medications over many years to treat a hormone insufficiency. She had no complaints involving the vulva.

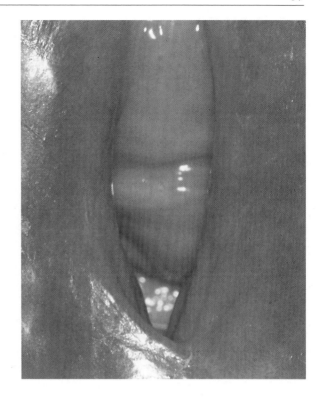

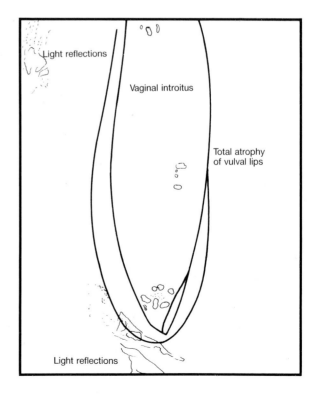

**Fig. 4.52: Vulval dystrophy
(previously known as
kraurosis vulvae)
with secondary leukoplakia**

Patient: 67 years old. An area
of whitish, thick, hyperkeratotic squamous epithelium appears well demarcated from
the somewhat atrophic and
pinkish epidermis of the vulva.
The patient had no symptoms,
but the presence of leukoplakia necessitates regular
checkups every 6 months.

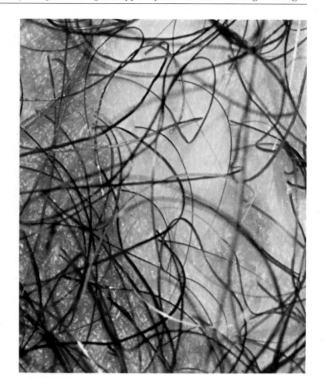

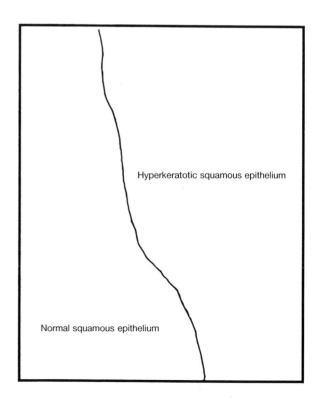

Hyperkeratotic squamous epithelium

Normal squamous epithelium

**Fig. 4.53: Vulval dysplasia
with coarse leukoplakia
(Morbus Bowen)**

Patient: 29 years old. Scaly,
whitish plaques, clearly elevated from the vulval epithelium are observed near the
vaginal fourchette. Contrast
with Fig. 4.52, in which the
whitish patches are even with
the vulval epithelial surface.
This patient had presented 5
years previously with coarse
leukoplakia of the cervix, and
a hysterectomy was per-
formed. At this time the atypical epithelial area was totally
excised.
Histology: carcinoma in situ —
Morbus Bowen.

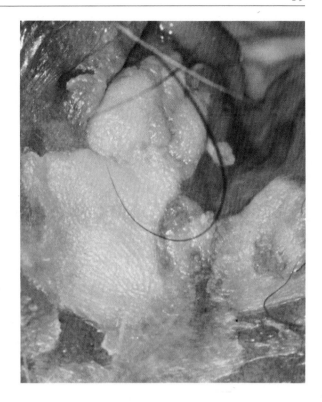

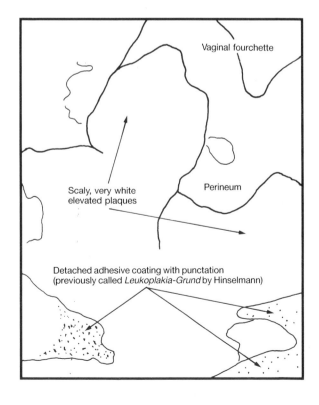

Vaginal fourchette

Scaly, very white
elevated plaques

Perineum

Detached adhesive coating with punctation
(previously called *Leukoplakia-Grund* by Hinselmann)

Fig. 4.54: Severe vulval dystrophy

Patient: 52-year-old para 2. Longstanding atrophic changes. The finding lichen sclerosus et atrophicus with secondary leukoplakia was histologically confirmed.

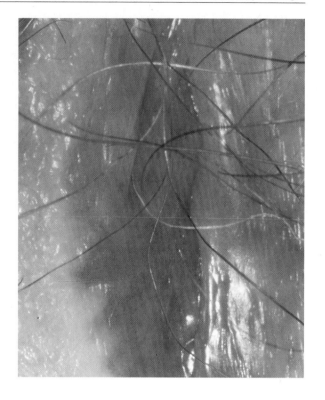

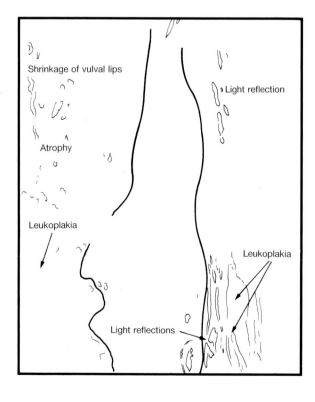

Shrinkage of vulval lips

Light reflection

Atrophy

Leukoplakia

Leukoplakia

Light reflections

Fig. 4.55: Angiokeratoma (benign teleangiectasia)

Patient: 37-year-old para 3. A cherry-sized superficial ulcerative nodule is seen to the right of the vulva. Extensive excision of the surrounding healthy tissue is always mandatory to ensure total removal of a possible melanoma. The patient had no symptoms.

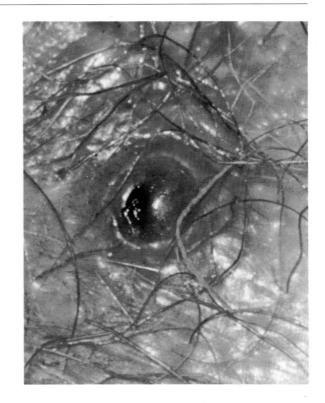

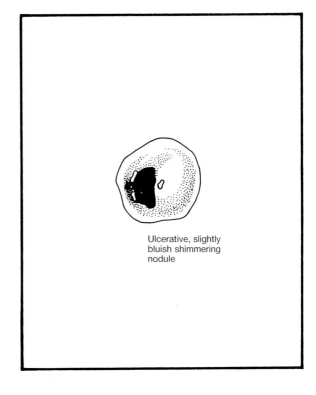

Ulcerative, slightly bluish shimmering nodule

Fig. 4.56: Pea-sized, bluish nodules near the labium majus; histologically a melanoma

Patient: 64 years old. The patient is postmenopausal with a recently discovered painful tumor.

Histologic findings: ulcerated nodular malignant melanoma of the labium majus. Level IV, depth of growth 1.5 mm.

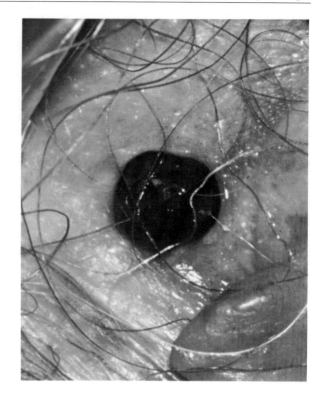

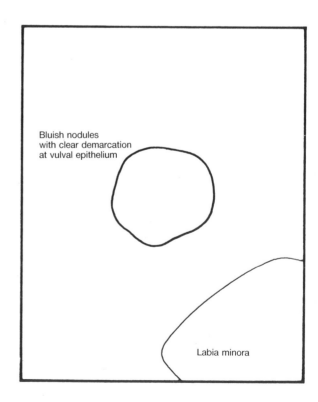

Bluish nodules with clear demarcation at vulval epithelium

Labia minora

Fig. 4.57: Appearance 3 months after tumor excision (See also Fig. 4.56)

Uneventful scar formation, without irritation. Regular checkups over 4 years have given no sign of recurrence or metastasis.

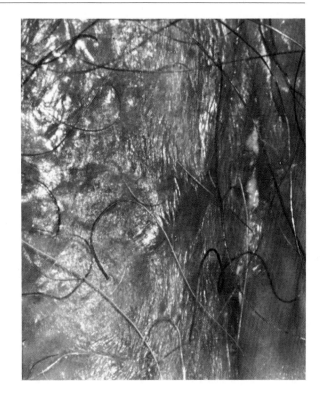

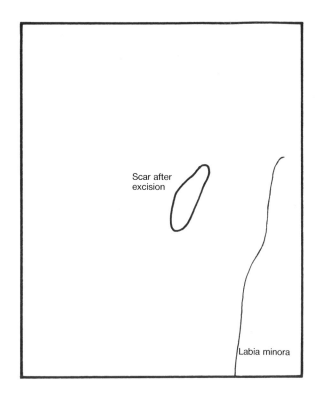

Scar after excision

Labia minora

4.2.8 Erosion

True erosion is defined by the presence of a genuine epithelial defect. Colposcopically exposed, easily bleeding stromal tissue is visible. HAMPERL explains this defect as being caused by a loss of squamous epithelium subsequent to inflammation or maceration by the irritating cervical mucus.

Histologically, the base of such an erosion shows a granulation tissue, which is often infiltrated by an inflammatory process. Particular attention has to be paid to the edge of an erosion to ascertain whether there is a flat or damlike border with vascularization.

The cause of an erosion is usually traumatic, for example in the course of delivery or speculum insertion. The latter is especially likely in older patients. Often the detached squamous epithelium can still be identified at the edge, and the experienced colposcopist will immediately diagnose the benign nature of this lesion. Erosions and even large ulcerations may also occur as a result of coital injuries. According to MESTWERDT and WESPI, pregnancy with its inherent epithelial hyperemia and vulnerability predisposes to this type of epithelial damage. Moreover, decubital erosions can develop in old patients wearing intravaginal ring pessaries for prolapse. Erosions caused by specific infections (tuberculosis, syphilis) are rather uncommon.

It is important to realize that both erosion and ulceration may represent the early stage of a malignant epithelial process. It is therefore mandatory to order histologic evaluation, even in the presence of a negative cytologic (Papanicolaou) smear, if local therapy of 3 to 4 weeks' duration has not healed the lesion. The malignancy index is given at approximately 11% in the literature. I consider this rather high, as explained below.

Without a colposcope the examiner is not able to differentiate between true erosion, ectopy, and transformation zone. Usually only a red spot or patch is visible, and this is wrongly termed erosion. As I mentioned previously, the use of 3% acetic acid during colposcopy is mandatory. Only after application will it be possible to identify the epithelial defect at the exposed reddened stromal tissue and to interpret the changes at the bordering squamous epithelium.

Classification remains difficult, however. International nomenclature continues to place this condition under the heading "various findings" and I have conformed to that usage. The reader is referred to the earlier discussion of this point. If the erosion is flat, the edges are smooth, and no atypical vascularization is visible, the findings can be considered unsuspicious. However, if there is an ulcer with elevated edge and atypical vessels, the finding is definitely suspicious and a biopsy is mandatory. See section 4.3.7 "Exophytic Changes – Ulcer".

Fig. 4.2.8 Erosion   95

Fig. 4.58: Erosion

Patient: 44 years old. Several erosions present at the posterior cervical lip. The squamous epithelium is detached from its base, leaving only remnants visible at the edges. The acute lesions in this patient have to be considered an artefact, possibly caused by speculum insertion. Colposcopic followup examinations indicated good healing of the defects.

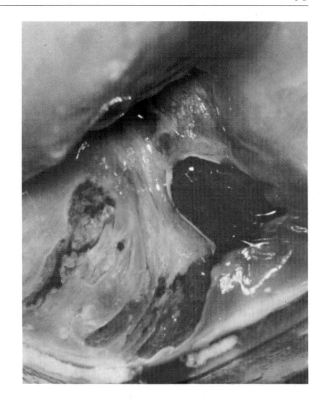

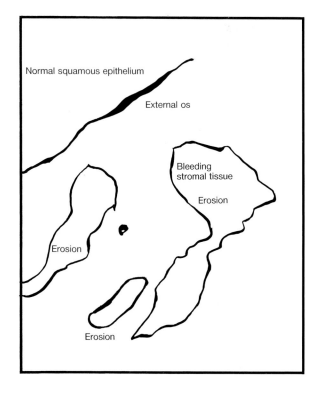

Fig. 4.59: Erosion

Patient: 60 years old, post-menopausal. An epithelial defect with loss of squamous epithelium has developed. Marked vascularization of the underlying tissue may be clearly recognized. These findings were observed on the right side of the vaginal vault near the cervix during a routine examination. The patient had no symptoms. Patients exhibiting such changes must regularly undergo careful evaluation. In this case, the lesion healed quickly after local estrogen therapy (See Fig. 4.60).

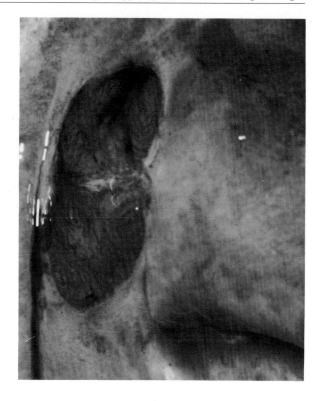

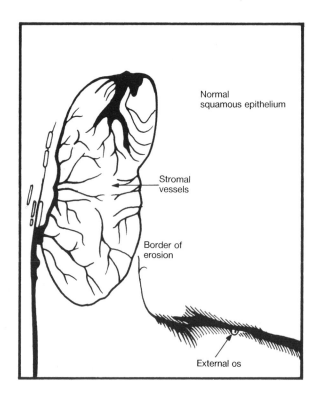

Fig. 4.2.8 Erosion   97

Fig. 4.60: Scar formation; appearance after local estrogen treatment of an erosion (See also Fig. 4.59)

Patient: Same as in Fig. 4.59, 3 weeks after local estrogen treatment. A distinct scar is observed to the right of the vaginal vault. Another minor tissue defect is visible in the upper left-hand corner, close to 10 o'clock.

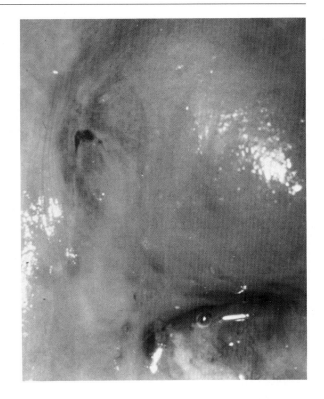

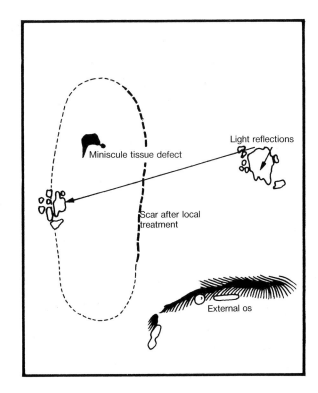

Fig. 4.61: Erosion; decubital ulcer (total procidentia)

Patient: 80-year-old wearer of ring pessary. Such lesions are more commonly seen in old patients who have worn ring pessaries for several years. There is an easily visible border to the neighboring squamous epithelium, which shows early keratosis. A yellowish stroma containing blood vessels appears inside the ulcer.

As for all erosive lesions the rule to be applied is: If healing is not achieved by local medication, histologic examination is mandatory.

This patient was treated by cervical amputation and subtotal colpocleisis (method according to LABHARDT).

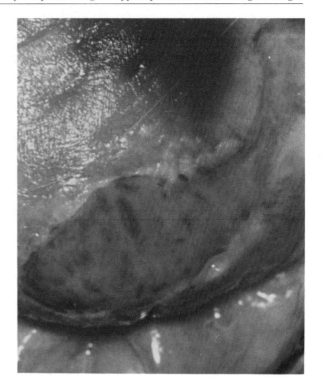

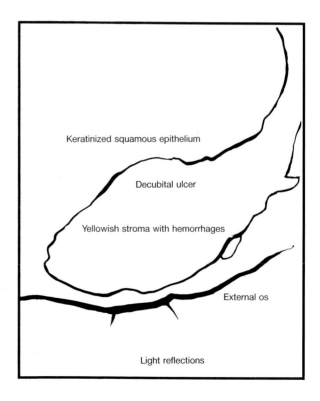

Keratinized squamous epithelium

Decubital ulcer

Yellowish stroma with hemorrhages

External os

Light reflections

Fig. 4.2.8 Erosion 99

Fig. 4.62: Erosion; decubital ulcer

Patient: 81-year-old pessary wearer. Here, too, one clearly recognizes hypervascular stromal tissue and a distinct demarcating edge to the squamous epithelium. The extensive erosive area was treated after the pessary was removed. The lesion healed completely and a soft plastic intrauterine device was again inserted.

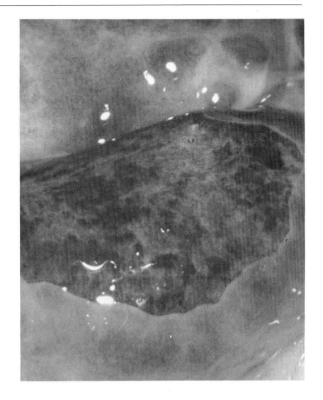

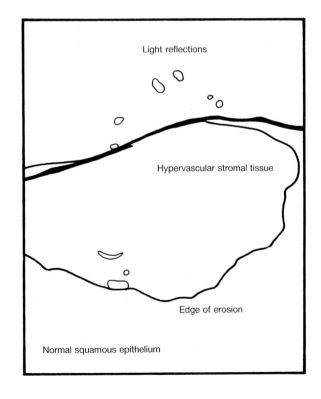

Fig. 4.63: Erosion; small ulcerations at the vaginal vault following hysterectomy

Patient: 44 years old. This patient developed these small, easily bleeding epithelial defects as a result of coital injury. The lesions healed within a short time after local therapy.

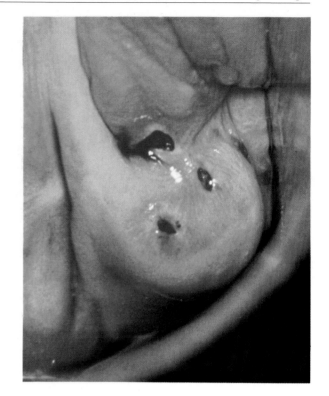

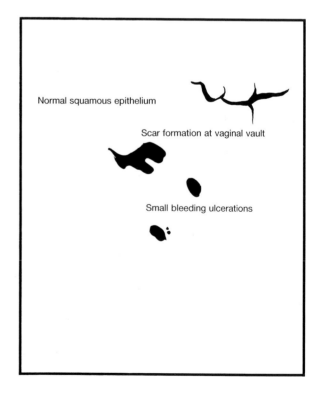

Normal squamous epithelium

Scar formation at vaginal vault

Small bleeding ulcerations

4.2.9 Inflammation

In 33 years as a practicing gynecologist I have found a wide variety of inflammatory changes in the area of the cervix, vagina, and vulva. The literature reports an overall incidence of 30%, which I think is a little too high. Of 100 patients chosen randomly from my practice, 28% complained of vaginal discharge, 6% suffered from vaginitis, and 8% had vulvitis. The vagina and cervix promptly respond to infective agents by increased vascularization.

4.2.9.1 Vaginitis

In the presence of vaginitis the discharge contains a variety of microorganisms. A detailed description is beyond the scope of this atlas, but two forms of presentation should be differentiated: Diffuse vaginitis is characterized by pronounced uniform erythema of the epithelium, often accompanied by edema; no detail can be identified through the colposcope. The other type is punctation-like localized vaginitis with circumscribed areas of engorged vessels presenting either as multiple red dots or patches.

4.2.9.2 Cervicitis

Inflammation of the cervix leads to differing degrees of increased vascularization of the ectopy and transformation zone. Colposcopic interpretation is not always easy; the cytologist is similarly confronted with a puzzling situation when evaluating the cervical smear of a patient with infection. It is therefore a good principle to perform followup colposcopy after an adequate period of treatment.

The diagnosis of cervicitis can also be assumed if the cervical mucus loses its clear transparency and becomes turbid. The patient usually reports vaginal discharge and pain. Unfortunately, there are no unequivocal criteria differentiating between normal cervical epithelium and an inflammatory process. Sometimes the absence of a sharp demarcation line may indicate the benign nature of the findings. The Schiller test is also not of any help in these cases since an inflamed surface can be iodine-negative, as can atypical epithelium.

4.2.9.3 Vulvitis

In the discussion of inflammatory changes, vulvitis needs to be mentioned briefly. The vulva shows edema and redness, and the affected area can be quite painful. The infection may occur secondarily to cervicitis and vaginitis.

4.2.9.4 Causes of Inflammation

There are numerous reasons for the inflammatory reaction. Systemic infection is a possible cause, as are mechanical and traumatic factors (coitus, vaginal douches, ring pessaries, etc.). Most important are the microorganisms such as bacteria, fungi, and *Trichomonas*. Inflammatory changes have also been reported to originate from an allergic reaction, for example, following the use of drugs or cosmetic agents. Finally, estrogen deficiency belongs to the list of causes as a contributing factor in the development of genital inflammation. Further details are described in section 4.2.10.

Fig. 4.64: Severely inflamed polypoid ectopy undergoing metaplasia

Patient: 22-year-old, 8 weeks postpartum. Such proliferative changes will be encountered, as repeatedly demonstrated, during and after pregnancy, but also in women taking oral contraceptives. If secondary infection is present, as in this case, assessment of the colposcopic appearance may prove difficult.

Treatment should be instigated first, followed by repeat colposcopy. The lesion in this patient healed completely after cauterization using Semm's coagulator (See also Fig. 4.65).

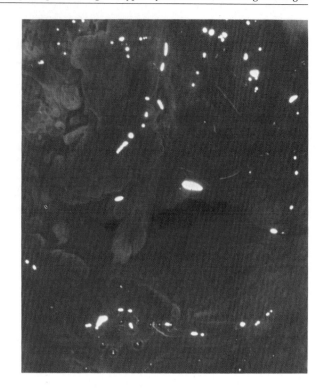

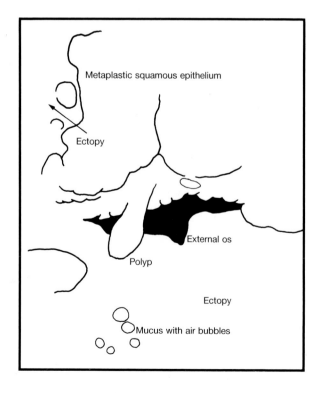

Fig. 4.65: Cervical appearance after two cauterizations

Patient: Same as in Fig. 4.64. The inflammatory changes healed completely after cauterization was performed twice using the Semm's coagulator.

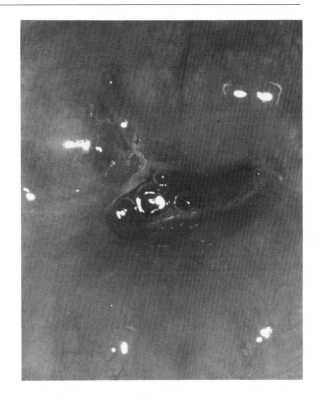

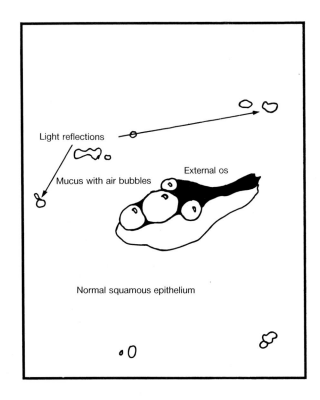

Fig. 4.66: Inflammation;
***Trichomonas* vaginitis**

Patient: 30-year-old   with
vaginal discharge and severe
inflammation.   Diffuse   vascularization demonstrating a
punctation-like pattern at the
anterior and posterior cervical
lips. A few of the vessels appear to some extent atypical
(bizarre   and   fragmented
shapes). Details can be recognized only with difficulty.
This patient had a *Tricho-*
monas vaginalis infection.

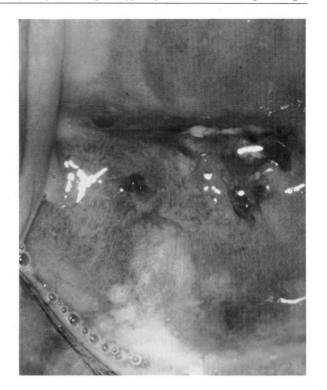

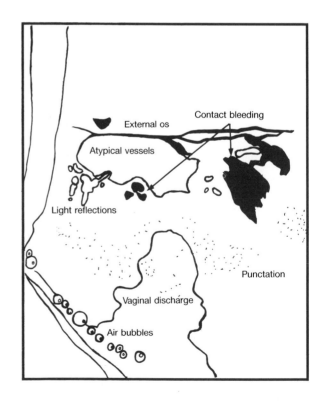

Fig. 4.67: Inflammation; *Trichomonas* vaginitis

Patient: 46 years old. The vaginal vault shows an inflammatory, mainly punctation-like vascular pattern. This patient had a previous hysterectomy and now presented with a pronounced infection due to *Trichomonas vaginalis.*

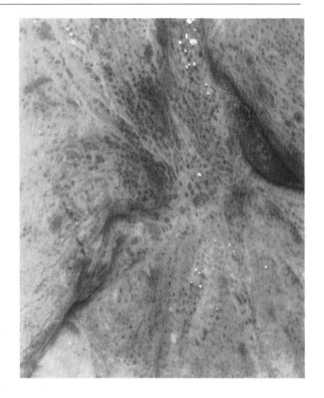

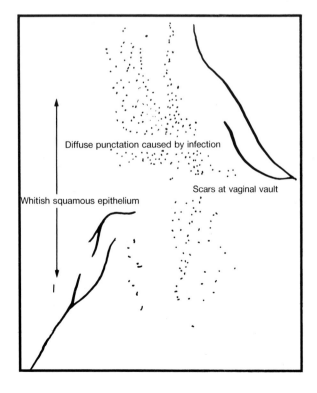

Diffuse punctation caused by infection

Scars at vaginal vault

Whitish squamous epithelium

Fig. 4.68: Inflammation; acute *Trichomonas* vaginitis

According to the reliable report of the patient, severe itching and burning sensations of the vagina developed after a spa visit. The vagina appears extremely swollen with a plaquelike structure. The grayish-white mucoid discharge visible in the crypts was even more pronounced before the application of 3% acetic acid. The symptoms disappeared quickly upon local treatment.

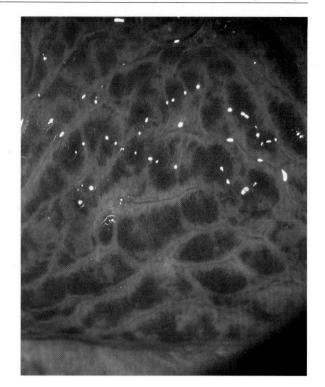

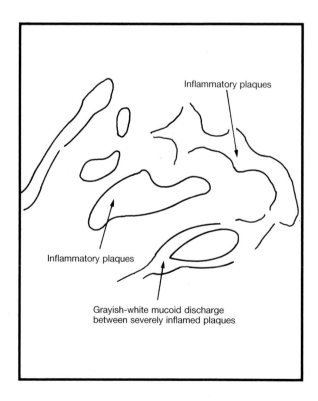

Inflammatory plaques

Inflammatory plaques

Grayish-white mucoid discharge between severely inflamed plaques

Fig. 4.69: Diffuse vaginitis

Patient: 50 years old. The cervical and vaginal surfaces demonstrate a marked redness. A diffuse, fine punctation pattern can be seen consisting of distinct red spots which correspond to the tips of stromal papillae with their capillary loops (WESPI).
The patient suffered from *Trichomonas vaginitis.*

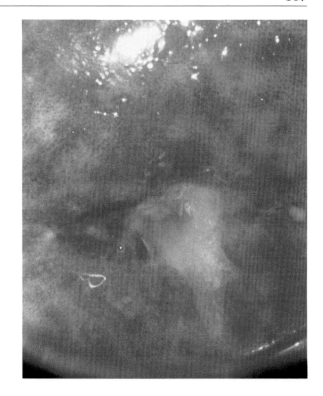

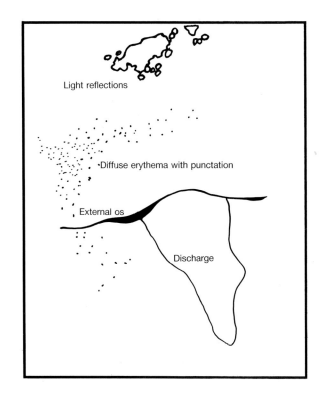

Light reflections

Diffuse erythema with punctation

External os

Discharge

Fig. 4.70: Inflammation; vaginal discharge due to *Candida* infection

Patient: 38-year-old para 2 with an IUD in place. Strong, whitish, brittle vaginal discharge is due to *Candida* infection. Here, too, the lesion healed completely after therapy.

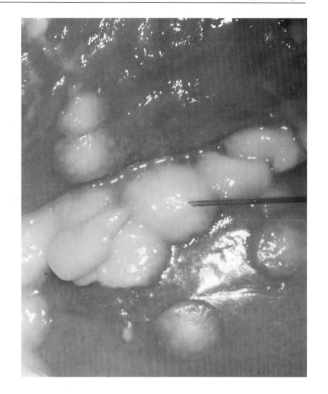

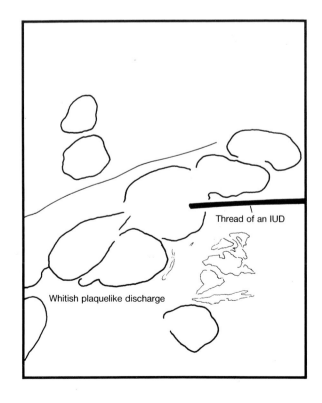

Thread of an IUD

Whitish plaquelike discharge

Fig. 4.71: Mosaic; inflammation

Patient: 22-year-old on oral contraceptives. A tongue-shaped area of fine mosaic extends anteriorly to the posterior cervical lip. The external os is centrally surrounded by columnar ectopy.

This patient on oral contraceptives had vaginal discharge due to *Candida* infection. A whitish patchy discharge is present on the cervical surface at 12 o'clock and on the lateral vaginal walls. These signs suggest a fungal contamination even on macroscopic inspection. Such fine mosaic, as well as fine punctation structures, is often observed in inflammatory processes. The slightly coarse and somewhat irregular surface structure is caused by the proliferative stimulation of oral contraceptives.

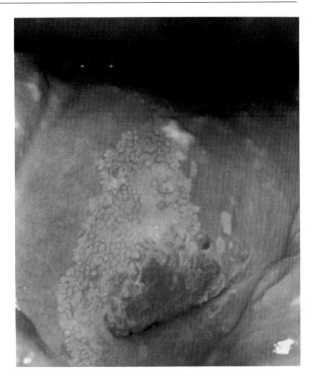

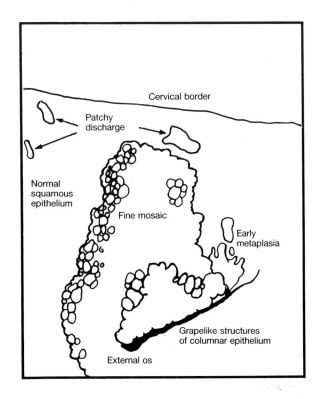

Fig. 4.72: Erosion with severe inflammation

Patient: 33-year-old taking oral contraceptives for 2 years. Rather widespread hemorrhagic erosions are observed on the edge of the posterior cervical lip. Squamous epithelial growth is seen beginning at the edge and extending toward the external os. Individual details are not visible because of the severe inflammation.

The same thing applies here as previously stated: A followup colposcopic evaluation after the inflammation has been treated is mandatory. And further, histologic assessment is necessary if the erosion is not healed.

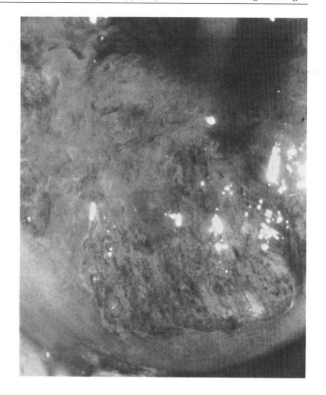

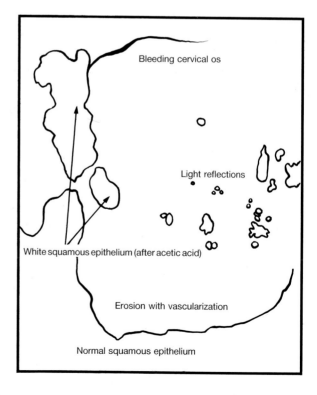

Fig. 4.73: Severe, erosive inflammation of the cervix

Patient: 27-year-old nullipara. Such severe inflammatory reactions with areas of true erosion, covered in part by polypoid mucous plaque and darkish hemorrhaging and necrosis, are rarely seen. The findings resemble those seen after chemical cauterization. The patient had developed an allergic reaction after using a hygienic spray; this may have contributed to the occurrence of the severe inflammation. In such a case colposcopic evaluation is not possible. Local therapy is indicated followed by colposcopic reevaluation.

Histologic findings: True erosion with pronounced, partly granulomatous inflammatory reaction.

The lesion healed completely after local therapy.

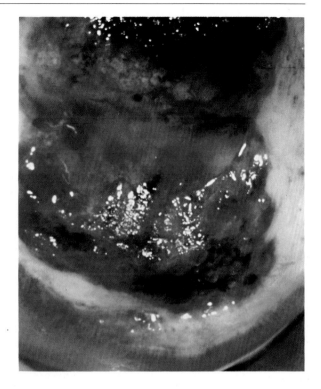

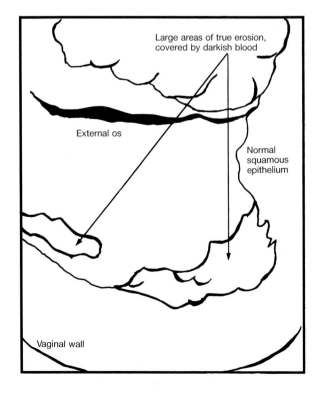

Large areas of true erosion, covered by darkish blood

External os

Normal squamous epithelium

Vaginal wall

Fig. 4.74: Acute diffuse vaginitis (See also Fig. 4.75)

Patient: 68 years old. The vaginal and cervical surfaces are red and edematous, and the epithelium tends to bleed easily on contact.

The patient reported dyspareunia and postcoital bleeding. Estrogen deficiency most probably contributed to the occurrence of this condition. The symptoms ceased after local application of an estrogenic compound.

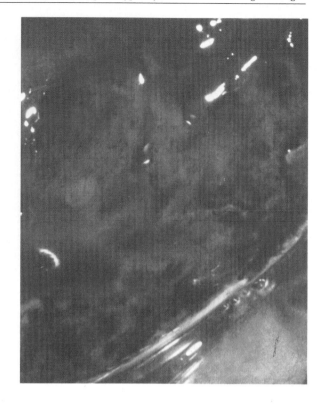

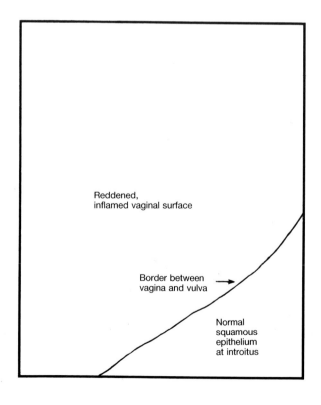

Reddened, inflamed vaginal surface

Border between vagina and vulva →

Normal squamous epithelium at introitus

Fig. 4.75: Cervical appearance after local estrogen therapy for vaginitis

Patient: Same as in Fig. 4.74. The red inflammatory reaction has disappeared. The vaginal epithelium appears normal again, and the 68-year-old patient had no further symptoms.

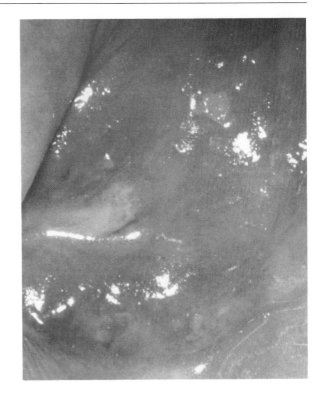

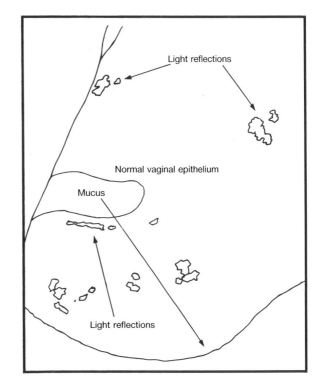

4.2.10 Atrophic Changes

Atrophic changes of the vulva, vagina, and cervix usually occur when ovarian function has ceased, mainly after menopause. In sexually mature women, atrophic changes are always an indication of systemic secretory disturbances. Such findings are seen in patients with primary sterility, but also in those with hypoplasia, ovarian insufficiency, or abnormal ovarian function.

According to HAMPERL, atrophy develops when the cells absorb less nutritional material, leading to a reduction in size, loss of protoplasm, and shrinkage of the nucleus. Apart from the diminished supply of nutrition, cells can also atrophy with age; the condition is then known as senile atrophy. A third possibility is atrophy due to inactivity. Finally, pressure atrophy can be caused purely by mechanical cellular damage.

This discussion deals mainly with senile atrophy. When ovarian function ceases, estrogens are no longer available for the maturation of the epithelium. In particular the upper layer of superficial cells may disappear completely. The epithelium, now consisting mainly of basal and parabasal cells, becomes very thin, the small vessels beneath becoming discernible. The insufficiently matured epithelium produces no glycogen, and the normal protective acidity of the vagina is lost. Secondary infection often follows (See section 4.2.9.)

The atrophic epithelium tends to be sensitive and can easily be damaged. Colposcopically it presents with a variety of changes: Spotty bleeding can be seen adjacent to diffuse hemorrhages and small erosions. Vessels appear as reddish dots resembling fine punctation. This condition may lead to diagnostic difficulties because it differs only minimally from the true punctation seen within atypical epithelium, which is generally harmless. Atrophic changes usually disappear quickly after topical application of estrogen, eventually supplemented with orally administered estrogens and antiinflammatory agents.

The healing process can readily be observed by photographic documentation of the colposcopic findings.

Fig. 4.76.: Atrophic epithelium

Patient: 53-year-old para 2. Thinning of the squamous epithelium is indicated by a pinkish color tone and the appearance of easily discernible vessels, particularly at the anterior cervical lip.

Such atrophic changes, not causing any symptoms as in this case, are found in women during and after menopause when estrogen production ceases. This patient had a dimplelike shrinkage of the external cervical os.

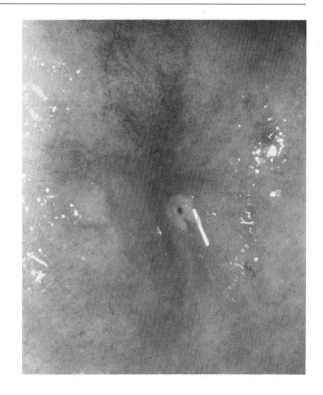

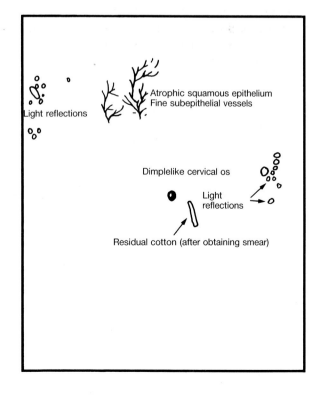

Fig. 4.77: Multiple hemorrhagic foci with atrophy

Patient: 65 years old, postmenopausal. Owing to atrophy, the squamous epithelium is so thin that even minimal contact or touching is immediately followed by hemorrhage of the fragile subepithelial vessels.

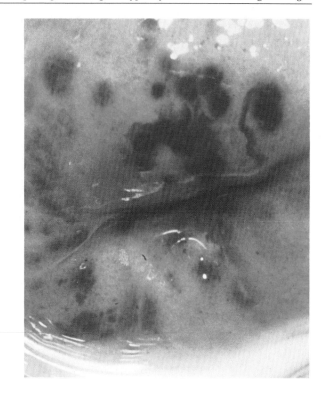

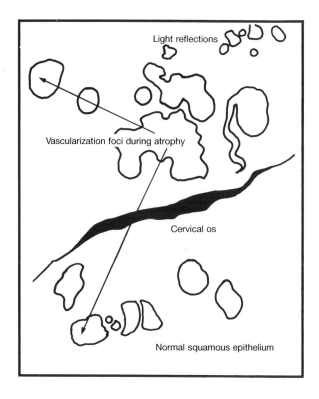

Fig. 4.78: Atrophic epithelium with multiple vascularized foci

Patient: 70 years old. The multiple vascularized foci at the posterior cervical lip are due to the fragility of the thin squamous epithelium. The anterior cervical lip shows more petechial bleeding foci. Furthermore, a small polyp covered by squamous epithelium is present at the external os.

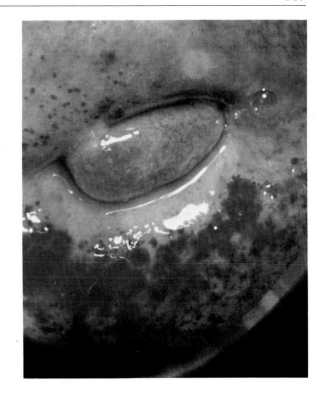

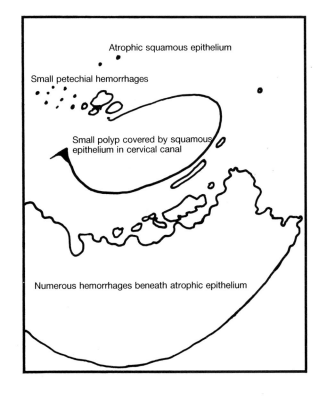

**Fig. 4.79: Atrophic
epithelium (See also
Fig. 4.80)**

Patient: 42-year-old nullipara
with primary sterility. Atrophic squamous epithelium
with two small tongue-shaped,
fine white areas (after acetic
acid application) between 2
and 4 o'clock – a sign of insufficient hormone function.

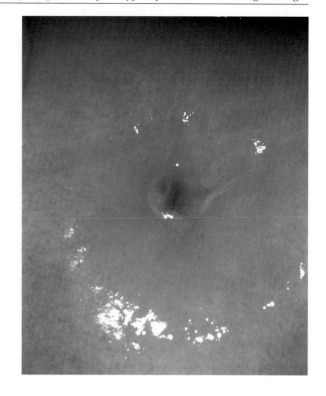

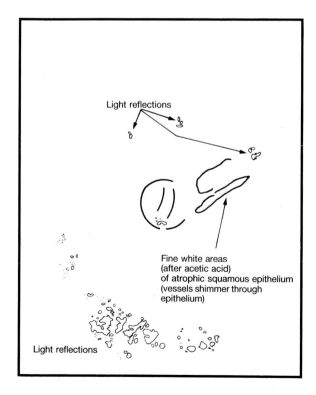

Fig. 4.80: Atrophic epithelium

Patient: Same as in Fig. 4.79, eleven years later. The atrophic area has expanded. Unsuspicious petechial foci are visible. An obvious, definitive sign of atrophy is also a certain dimplelike depression near the barely recognizable external os. The total observation time is 22 years.

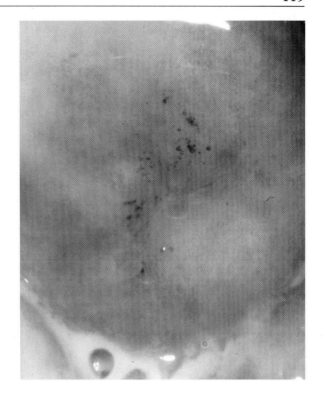

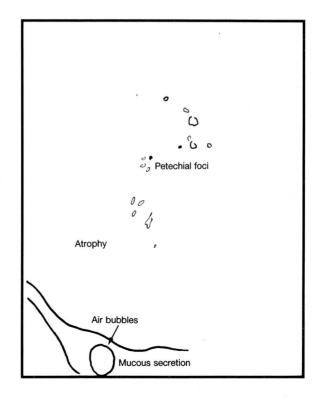

Fig. 4.81: Atrophic squamous epithelium

Patient: 20-year-old nullipara with uterine hypoplasia and secondary amenorrhea. The squamous epithelium is slightly atrophic. Faint oval area of fine white epithelial discolorization (after acetic acid application) around the external os permits distinct differentiation of the normal squamous epithelium. Such a distinct finding in a young patient is a sign of systemic secretory disturbance.

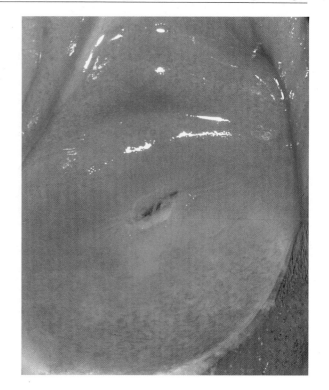

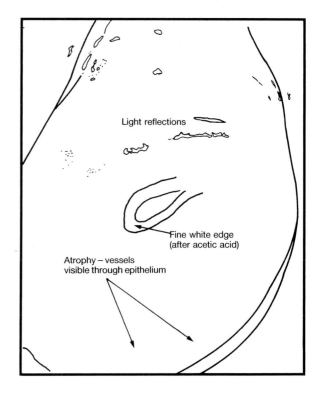

4.3 Atypical (Abnormal) Colposcopic Findings

4.3.1 Iodine-negative Area

In this edition, as opposed to the second edition, I have categorized the iodine-negative findings as atypical (abnormal) findings. Schiller's iodine test has already been described (See section 2.2).

To repeat: I have found it unnecessary to use Schiller's test at each colposcopic examination since it is rather unspecific. Others have also reached this conclusion, but opinions differ greatly. There are authors who consider the method indispensable, believing there are "silent" iodine-negative areas that could be overlooked if Schiller's test is not done. I believe that all abnormal changes become clearly visible after the obligatory application of 3% acetic acid. Of course, the examiner should not be in a hurry and must allow enough time for the 3% acetic acid solution to act.

I have often stated that fine punctation, fine mosaic, and mucoid leukoplakia are histologically benign. Such epithelial changes, which HINSELMANN had referred to as atypical epithelium, are described as abnormal epithelium. They are classified

as colposcopic findings that do not require a biopsy.

It is known that inflamed as well as atrophic epithelium is often iodine-negative, which supports my point of view. As I already mentioned, abnormal or atypical epithelium can be very easily recognized after application of a 3% acetic acid solution. The negative Schiller's test is a valuable supportive method, however. In fact, prior to conization it is absolutely necessary to demarcate atypical epithelium. It is even more important to do so when taking biopsy specimens under colposcopic direction.

SCHILLER originally used the iodine test that was named after him for macroscopic observation of the cervix, and for this purpose it is indispensable. Today, however, no gynecologic examination can be considered thorough without a colposcopic evaluation. Should an iodine-negative area be found by a physician who does not do colposcopy, a colposcopic examination must be performed to clarify the findings.

I have not presented iodine-negative findings in a separate section but rather together with results after application of 3% acetic acid. (See Figs. 4.86, 4.88, 4.90, 4.99.)

4.3.2 Punctation

Now that the colposcopic term "punctation" has been internationally agreed upon, HINSELMANN's term (ground structure) has been dropped from the German nomenclature.

There are two different types of punctation: fine and coarse. *Fine punctation* is usually harmless and is characterized by the appearance of several reddish dots which correspond to the tips of stromal papillae and their capillary loops (WESPI). These reddish spots become visible when light falls on the terminal vessels as they form a loop almost at the surface of each stromal papilla. Fine punctation occurs most often in young women with ovarian insufficiency and in cases of atrophy. It may also be seen in some patients using oral contraceptives and in the presence of inflammation and viral infections. As pointed out, these changes are usually benign and they only require regular colposcopic and cytologic followup.

In contrast, *coarse punctation,* previously called "papillary ground structure," must always be viewed with suspicion. A biopsy should be performed even if the cytologic (Papanicolaou) smear is negative. WESPI gives the following description of coarse punctation:

> "The epithelium frequently has a glassy, yellowish appearance with small elevations, exhibiting dilated and pathological capillary loops in their centers. This finding indicates an early exophytic growth pattern which is almost typical for beginning carcinoma."

Like other atypical changes, coarse punctation is often sharply demarcated from normal epithelium. The assessment of the lesion becomes difficult when it extends into the endocervical canal. In such cases histologic examination should always be performed.

The incidence of punctation according to COUPEZ and associates lies between 0.8 and 2.75%; the probability of malignancy in these cases is 8%.

4.3.3 Mosaic

The earlier German term *Felderung,* coined by HINSELMANN, has also been replaced. The internationally accepted term is now *mosaic.*

As in punctation and leukoplakia, a distinction is made between fine and coarse mosaic, and the same remarks are valid for fine mosaic as for fine punctation. *Fine mosaic* is a harmless atypical finding that occasionally can be seen in adolescent females with ovarian insufficiency, but also in the presence of inflammation, with viral infections, and in women taking oral contraceptives. The lesion is characterized by the occurrence of larger or smaller fields with round, rhombic, or tetragonal shapes that are separated by fine red lines. According to GLATTHAAR, these fields correspond histologically to thickened epithelium that has a whitish appearance because of its minimal transparency. These epithelial proliferations often develop in cervical crypts within a transformation zone. The red demarcation lines are caused by stromal ridges which connect the stromal papillae and contain vessels running parallel to the surface. GANSE describes the development of mosaic as a masonry-like growth of atypical epithelium whereby numerous individual blocks create a mosaic pattern on the surface.

Coarse mosaic has a papillomatous elevation above the surface contour. The red demarcation lines are capillaries. These may be thickened and pronounced or may even show a highly irregular course. Another form was previously described as concave *Felderung.* The coarse mosaic presents as a hollowing or a dentlike depression with a red border. This form is relatively rare; it is found mostly in atypical transformation zones (see section 4.3.5). The irregularity of the surface contour can best be seen by stereoscopic photography. Such findings should arouse suspicion and require histologic assessment, even if the cytologic smear is negative.

The incidence of coarse mosaic found during colposcopy is 2.9 to 3.2% according to COUPEZ and associates, who report a 7.1% probability of malignancy.

Fig. 4.82: Fine punctation

Patient: 19-year-old taking oral contraceptives. There is a tonguelike area on the anterior cervical lip with sharp demarcation from the neighboring normal epithelium. In the region of the external os it becomes an ectopy undergoing metaplasia. Such findings are commonly seen in young patients with ovarian insufficiency or in the presence of inflammation. They are usually harmless.

This 19-year-old patient, who was taking oral contraceptives, became infected with *Trichomonas vaginalis.* The cytologic (Papanicolaou) smear proved negative and, after treatment of the *Trichomonas* infection, further management was conservative. Regular followup examinations were performed at 6-month intervals. Ten years later, the colposcopic findings were unchanged, and numerous Papanicolaou smears taken over that period have been negative.

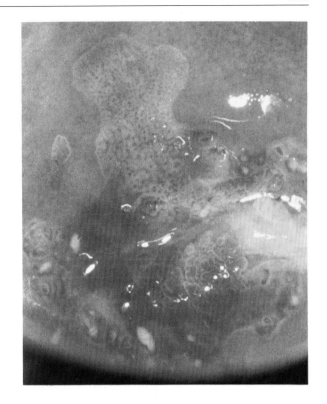

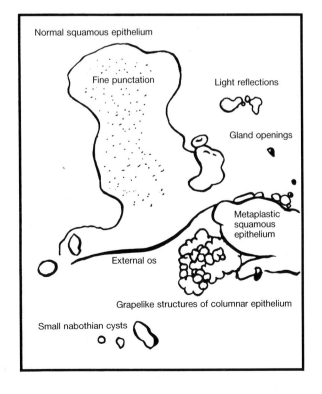

Fig. 4.83: Fine punctation/ fine mosaic

Patient: 39 years old. A tongue-shaped, fine white (after acetic acid application) epithelial area of punctation is seen at the anterior cervical lip. Fine mosaic is seen near the external os. In addition, several gland openings are visible between 12 and 1 o'clock, which is a certain sign that the transformation process has been completed.

If the cytologic (Papanicolaou) smears are negative, a checkup every 6 months is sufficient for this patient.

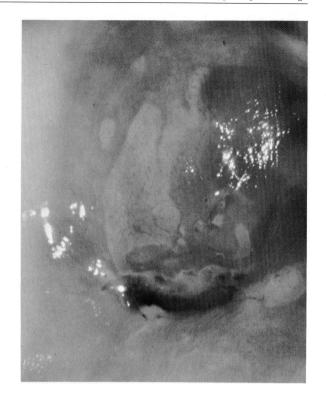

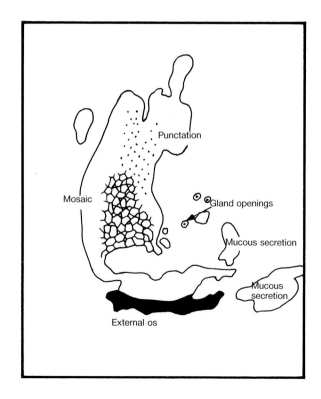

Fig. 4.84: Punctation

Patient: 31-year-old primipara. A sharply demarcated area of punctation is seen at the anterior cervical lip. The lesion is rather large and extends into the cervical canal. To some extent the punctation appears coarse, being slightly elevated above the normal surface. This primipara was treated by conization and curettage despite a negative cytologic (Papanicolaou) smear.

Histology: chronic inflammatory reaction of columnar ectopy with papillary mucosal hypertrophy and increased squamous epithelial regeneration with formation of stromal papillae and ridges (mild dysplasia – CIN I).

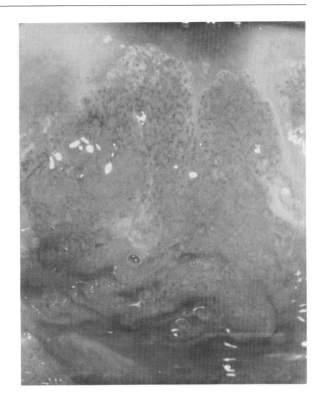

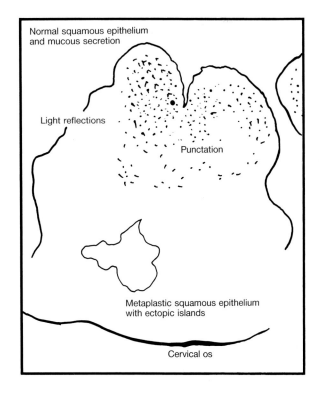

**Fig. 4.85: Fine mosaic
(See also Figs. 4.86, 4.87,
and 4.88)**

Patient: 26-year-old contraceptive user. Two areas of
fine mosaic are visible on the
anterior cervical lip and on the
right side of the external os.
After application of 3% acetic
acid some of the epithelium
has turned white. A further
finding is the small polyp at
the external os, which was
covered by mucus.

The patient has now been reg-
ulary examined for 18 years
(See Figs. 4.87 and 4.88). During this time no changes were
observed, and repeated cytologic (Papanicolaou) smears
have been negative. At the
time this colpophotograph was
taken, the patient was 26
years old and had used a
number of different contraceptives.

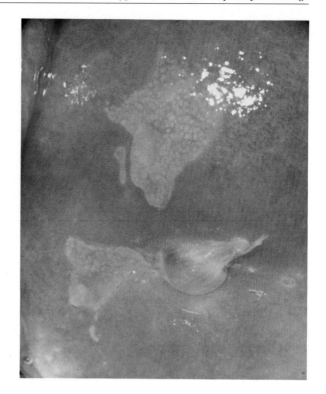

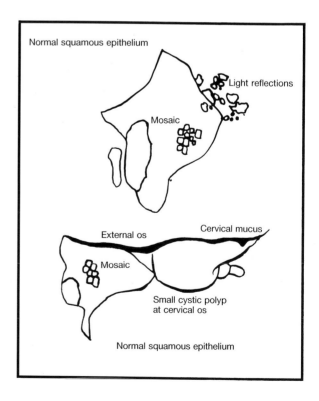

Fig. 4.86: Iodine-negative epithelial area

Patient: Same as in Fig. 4.85. After the application of iodine solution, the areas of fine mosaic are distinctly lighter than the rest of the epithelium. This is due to the lack of glycogen. In contrast, the normal epithelial cells take up a brown color tone. The Schiller test is a rather unspecific method, since it allows no detail to be recognized. (See section 2.2 and Figs. 4.85, 4.87, and 4.88).

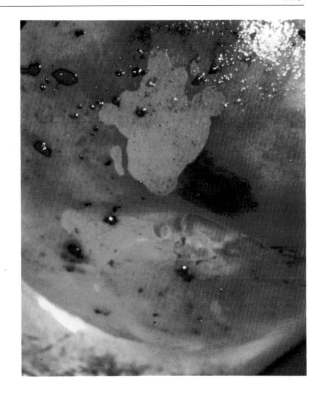

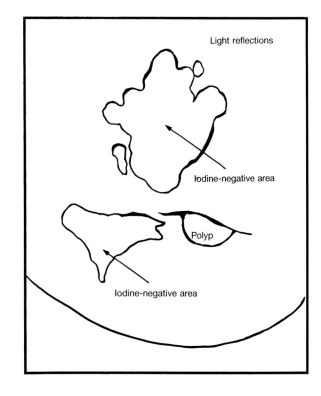

**Fig. 4.87: Fine mosaic
(See also Figs. 4.85, 4.86,
and 4.88)**

Patient: Same as in Figs. 4.85
and 4.86, 15 years later. The
small, fine tongue-shaped
mosaic patch within a white
epithelial area visible at the
cervical lip shows hardly any
change. Adjacent to this and at
9 o'clock is a sign of fine erosion with white epithelium.
The patient has since had an
intrauterine device inserted.

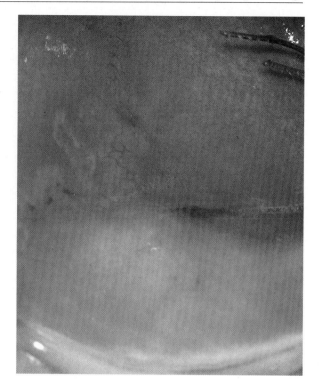

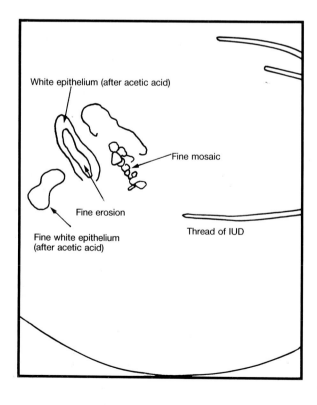

Fig. 4.88: Iodine-negative epithelial area

Patient: Same as in Fig. 4.85, 15 years later. After the application of iodine, a light tongue-shaped iodine-negative area is visible at the anterior cervical lip. In this case the mosaic structures can be recognized. (See also section 4.3.3).

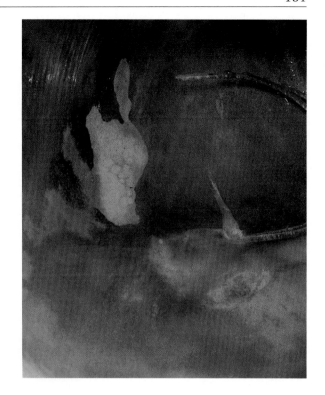

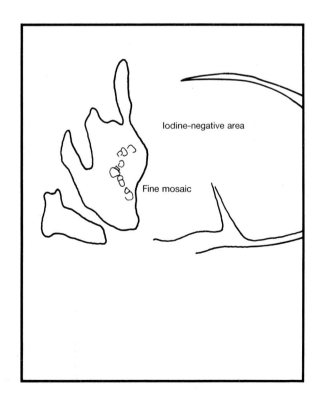

**Fig. 4.89: Mosaic
(See also Fig. 4.90)**

Patient: 46-year-old nullipara. Irregular, somewhat
coarse mosaic is visible on the
edge of the transformation
zone. The atypical epithelium
is raised from the normal surface level especially on the tip,
near the posterior cervical lip.
The difference is much more
easily recognizable in a three-
dimensional picture.
Histologic findings of a colposcopically directed punch
biopsy: moderate dysplasia –
CIN I.

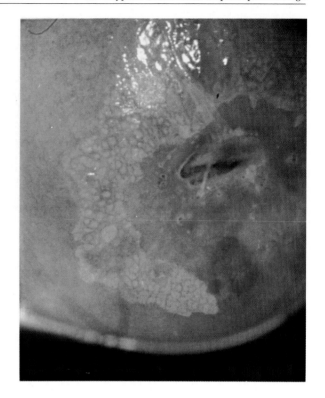

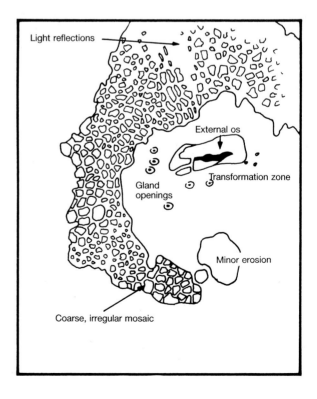

Fig. 4.90: Mosaic – iodine-negative area

Patient: Same as in Fig. 4.89. The atypical epithelium appears light brown after the application of iodine solution, while the normal squamous epithelium is stained dark brown. It is not possible to recognize any individual details, such as mosaic structures, after Schiller's iodine test has been done. (See the discussion of Schiller's test in section 2.2).

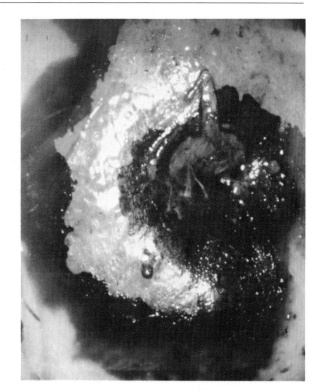

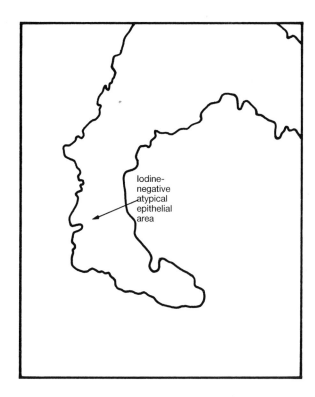

Iodine-negative atypical epithelial area

Fig. 4.91: Fine white epithelium with mosaic structure (See also Fig. 4.92)

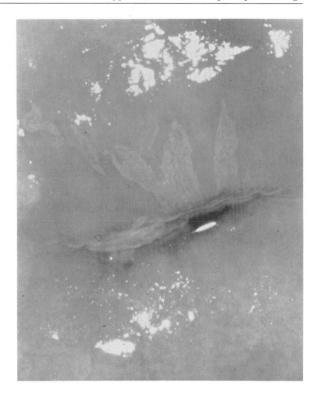

Patient: 43 years old; two spontaneous abortions, two normal deliveries. Several small fine tongue-shaped white (after acetic acid) epithelial areas with a hint of mosaic structures visible are seen at the anterior cervical lip. Numerous cytologic smears turned out negative. The extreme pale pink color of the mucosa reflects exactly that seen colposcopically. The paleness is probably due to a reduced blood circulation in the cervix. Physicians who frequently perform colposcopy will encounter such a finding regularly, although it is not common in the general population. For scientific purposes, a directed biopsy was taken and histologically evaluated: thickened superficial squamous epithelium, parakeratosis, squamous epithelial complexes growing into the aperture of mucosal glands.

This patient had had two normal deliveries and two miscarriages. A vaginal hysterectomy was performed because of uterine myomatosus.

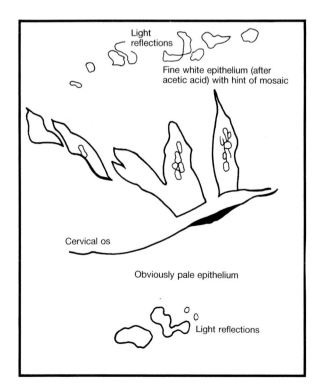

Fig. 4.92: Fine white epithelium with mosaic structure (See also Fig. 4.91)

Patient: Same as in Fig. 4.91 after 18 years. The fine, white, tonguelike mosaic area is still present at the anterior cervical lip, although noticeably smaller, and it now extends into the cervical canal.

There is some difficulty in classifying this finding. I had previously placed it under fine leukoplakia. The very slight white discolorization of the epithelium is recognizable even without the application of 3% acetic acid. The mosaic structures, on the other hand, are first distinctly visible after acetic acid has been applied. I therefore felt it more appropriate to classify the finding as under fine mosaic/fine white epithelium.

Today we know that such minor findings are also often seen with viral diseases of the cervix. The histologic assessment "parakeratosis" also is an indication of something that was not known at the time of the earlier examination.

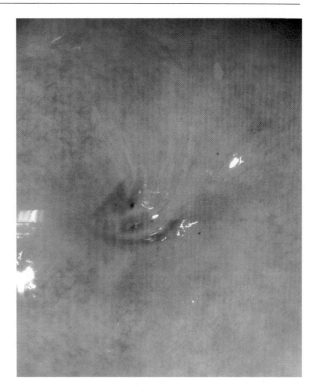

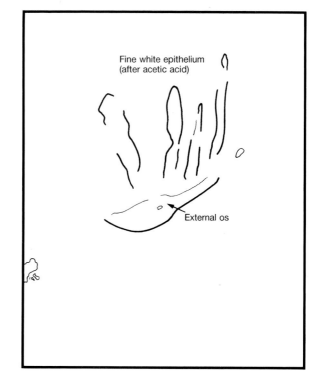

Fine white epithelium
(after acetic acid)

External os

Fig. 4.93: Coarse and irregular mosaic

Patient: 27-year-old nullipara. A large, somewhat irregular coarse mosaic with punched-out appearance is found on the edge of a polypoid transformation zone.

The proliferative epithelial changes seen centrally indicate the use of oral contraceptives. This finding was observed over 5 years, although the cytologic smear was negative. The Papanicolaou test was then group IV, the mosaic structures expanded, and the irregularity of the surface level became more pronounced. A comprehensive excision of the atypical epithelium followed after the area was identified by Schiller's iodine test.

Histology: moderate to severe dysplasia (CIN II to III). Complete regression of the atypical epithelium occurred after excision (observation time, 9 years). Repeated cytologic (Papanicolaou) smears were negative.

The patient has since had two normal deliveries. Because of the express wish of the then 27-year-old nullipara to have children, no further therapy was done. Regular annual colposcopic and cytologic checkups were considered sufficient. The last colposcopic finding: unsuspicious transformation zone.

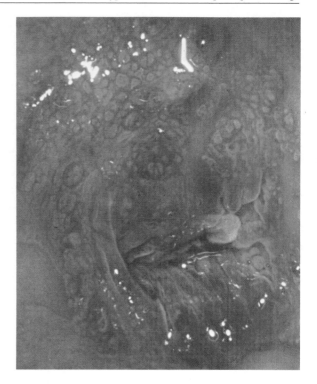

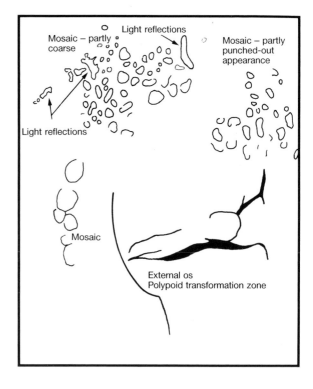

Fig. 4.94: Mosaic and punctation

Patient: 37-year-old gravida 3. A well demarcated area of slightly elevated punctation and irregular mosaic can be seen on the anterior cervical lip. The posterior lip exhibits an inflamed transformation zone. This type of finding would raise suspicion at the first examination, though one has to keep in mind that a severe infection is present.

A colposcopically directed punch biopsy was taken between 12 and 1 o'clock. Surprisingly, only mild dysplasia (CIN I) with a marked inflammatory reaction was found. Repeat Papanicolaou smears were cytologically negative.

On regular colposcopic followup examinations the atypical changes clearly reverted to normal. Thus, the severe concomitant inflammation very likely led to an overestimation of the colposcopic appearance. An important point from the history is that this patient had, in previous years, repeatedly received local treatment for vaginal discharge.

Further followup examinations are indicated.

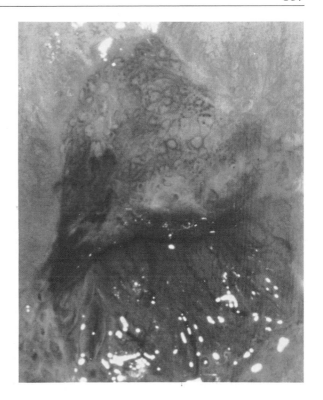

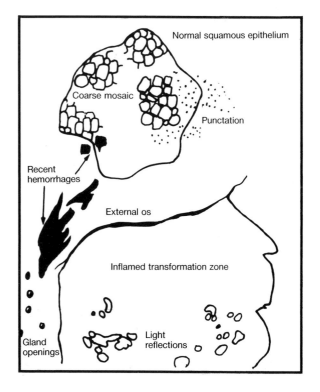

Fig. 4.95: Coarse punctation, coarse mosaic, polypoid transformation zone

Patient: 23-year-old primipara. A polypoid transformation zone on the anterior cervical lip contains areas of course mosaic and punctation. A demarcation line, separating the lesion from normal squamous epithelium, can clearly be seen in the upper portion, although it appears somewhat blurred laterally. The patient had been taking oral contraceptives and had experienced intermenstrual bleeding for the past 2 years. She had recently been treated for a *Candida* infection.

Histologic findings: carcinoma in situ (CIN III).

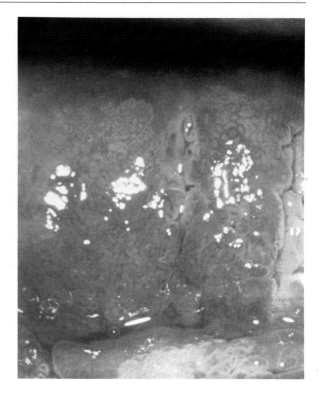

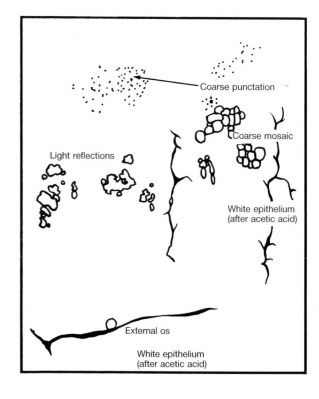

Fig. 4.96: Coarse punctation, coarse mosaic

Patient: 25 years old, 16 weeks pregnant. There is a large region of coarse mosaic in a white (after acetic acid) epithelial area. The atypical epithelium is distinctly elevated from the surface level, which is best seen in three-dimensional pictures. Note the thick red demarcation lines that separate the tissue fields creating the mosaic pattern. At other locations the atypical vessels cannot be so clearly differentiated. The posterior cervical lip is only partly visible and demonstrates a minor degree of epithelial atypia.

The cervical smear was falsely negative in this case, Papanicolaou II.

The patient was 16 weeks pregnant, and histologic evaluation was postponed. Cervical conization and curettage were performed after delivery, revealing the presence of carcinoma in situ (CIN III).

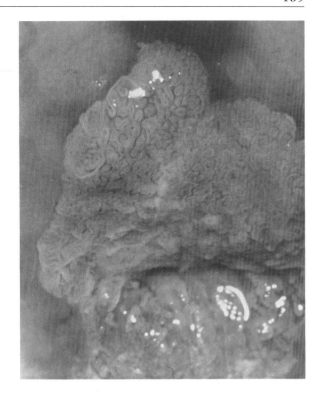

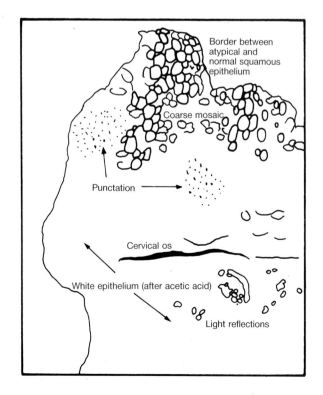

Fig. 4.97: Coarse mosaic, coarse punctation (See also Fig. 4.98)

Patient: 31 years old; one normal delivery, two spontaneous abortions. Before the application of 3% acetic acid, areas of mosaic alone are visible, and punctation cannot be easily identified. The whole region is diffusely reddened. Exact differentiation of the atypical epithelium becomes possible only after the use of acetic acid solution, as demonstrated in Fig. 4.98. The patient had been taking oral contraceptives for 8 years prior to the examination and had been treated for localized infection. Histology of a colposcopically directed punch biopsy: severe dysplasia – CIN III.
Cytologic findings: Papanicolaou smear positive, IV.
Therapy: cervical conization and curettage.

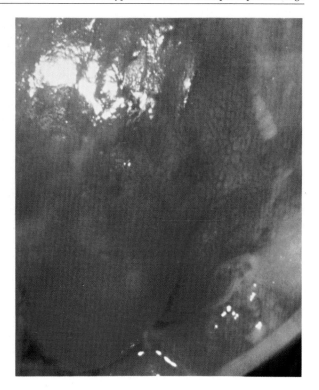

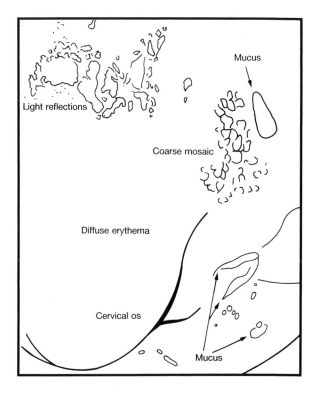

Fig. 4.98: Coarse mosaic, coarse punctation (See also Fig. 4.97)

Patient: same as in Fig. 4.97. The atypical epithelium becomes clearly visible only after application of 3% acetic acid. There is a sharp demarcation from the normal epithelium, especially visible at about 12 o'clock.
Hystologic findings: severe dysplasia – CIN III.
Therapy: cervical conization.

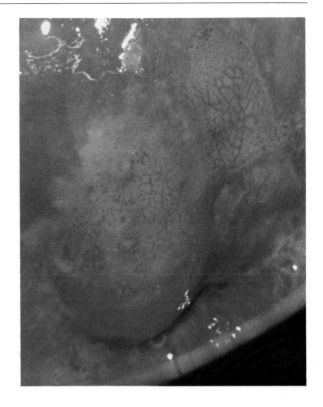

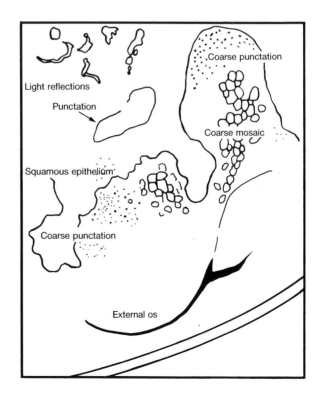

Fig. 4.99: Coarse, irregular mosaic, coarse punctation (See also Fig. 4.100)

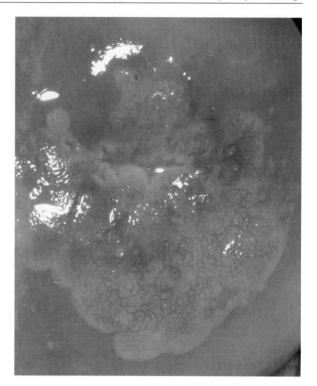

Patient: 30-year-old nullipara taking oral contraceptives. On the posterior cervical lip there is a relatively extended area of white epithelium with marked variation in the surface level as compared with the normal squamous epithelium. Coarse mosaic and coarse punctation are widespead within this area. The epithelium is stained intensely white, and the coloration is maintained. The atypical epithelium reaches farther to the right than is seen in this view. The border with the normal squamous epithelium is a sharp, damlike elevation, and the white coloring is particularly intense. The changed areas disappear on the right (on the viewer's left). In such cases, further photodocumentation is obviously necessary to present the border clearly in its entirety.

The patient is taking oral contraceptives, is a light smoker, and has had repeated fungal infections in the past and several sexual partners. The cytologic (Papanicolaou) smear is IVa. The atypical epithelial finding extends into the cervical canal, which makes it highly suspicious of carcinoma.

Histologic findings (conization): carcinoma in situ (CIN III − microcarcinoma); at one spot, even a breakthrough into the lymphatic system. Depth of growth is 2 mm.

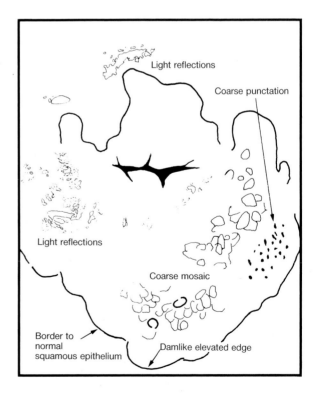

Fig. 4.100: Iodine-negative area (See also Fig. 4.99)

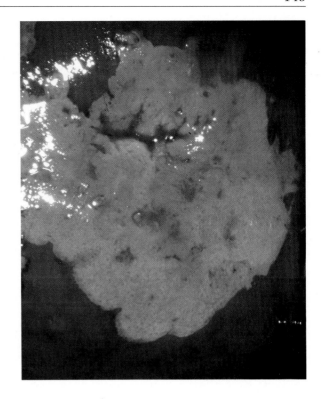

Patient: same patient as in Fig. 4.99. The entire large atypical epithelial area is iodine-negative. In this case, Schiller's test was of particular significance because a conization was performed, and for this the operator needed to differentiate clearly between atypical and normal (darkly brown-stained) squamous epithelium. Here, too, punctation and mosaic structures become invisible once iodine is applied. Further therapy was not planned in this special case. A hysterectomy was taken into consideration, but since the patient wanted very much to have children, this possibility was dropped for the time being. Regular cytologic and colposcopic check-ups (every 3 months) are necessary.

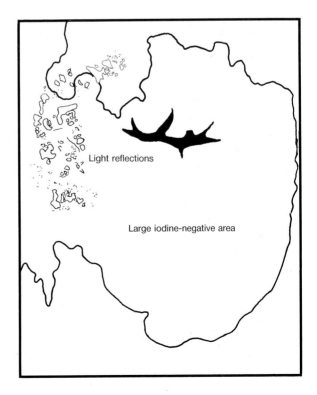

Light reflections

Large iodine-negative area

Fig. 4.101: Coarse punctation, irregular mosaic

Patient: 35-year-old primipara. A sharp demarcation between a larger atypical epithelium area and the normal epithelium. The edge shows a damlike elevation and is stained white by application of 3% acetic acid solution. Coarse punctation appears blotchlike and irregular next to individual irregular mosaic areas. The Papanicolaou smear is IV.
Histologic findings (conization): carcinoma in situ – CIN III.

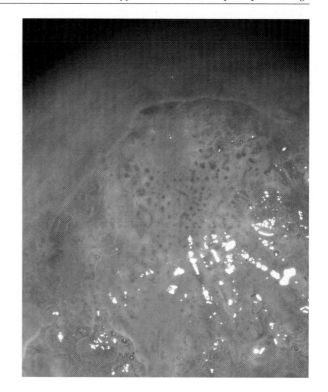

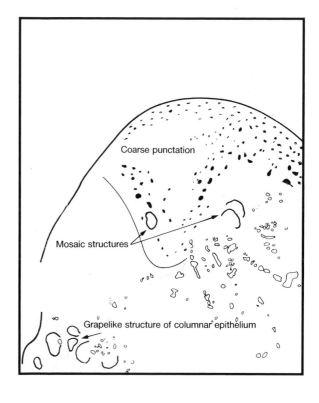

Coarse punctation

Mosaic structures

Grapelike structure of columnar epithelium

4.3.4 Leukoplakia

According to HINSELMANN, leukoplakia can be identified only through the colposcope. This may certainly be true for the smaller foci, but large areas of leukoplakia can easily be recognized with the unassisted eye. HINSELMANN regarded this epithelial lesion as premalignant, a conclusion that is too sweeping in view of our present knowledge. In 1932 my teacher, HASELHORST, made a valuable contribution to the subject by taking a more conservative and optimistic attitude. He advocated a thorough investigation with the colposcope, stating that "those colleagues not in possession of a colposcope have no excuse for withdrawing from the exploration of all matters concerning leukoplakia".

As with punctation and mosaic, a distinction must be made between fine (usually harmless) and coarse (always doubtful) leukoplakia. Colposcopically, leukoplakia appears as a white spot or patch. I think it is important to mention that leukoplakia is clearly recognizable without the application of 3% acetic acid solution, in contrast to white epithelium. Occasionally leukoplakia can be wiped away, revealing punctation, mosaic, or both. HINSELMANN therefore used the terms *Leukoplakiegrund* and *Leukoplakiefelderung.*

Fine leukoplakia is generally harmless. In most cases, histologic examination shows thickening of the squamous epithelium, known as *parakteratosis;* genuine keratinization (hyperkeratosis) is rare.

The value of colpophotographic documentation again becomes evident during followup examination of patients with leukoplakia. Comparing several pictures taken at different times allows the size and expansion of the lesion to be more readily assessed. Because of the lack of glycogen, the area will also be iodine-negative and sharply delineated from the rest of the epithelium. MESTWERDT and WESPI consider fine leukoplakia to be unimportant as regards malignancy.

Coarse leukoplakia is characterized by a flat, wartlike or papillomatous elevation above the level of the surrounding surface. Again, this type of lesion can be clearly observed by stereoscopic colpophotography. Coarse leukoplakia should always arouse suspicion and requires histologic assessment. This is best achieved by a colposcopically directed punch biopsy.

The incidence of leukoplakia according to HINSELMANN is 1.5%, which corresponds to the percentage given by COUPEZ and his coworkers (1–2%), whereas MESTWERDT found an occurrence of 4 to 6% in his cases. COUPEZ reports the lesion to be malignant in 4.9%, whereas BAJARDI and LIMBURG give the figure at 8 to 9%.

Fig. 4.102: Fine leukoplakia

Patient: 50-year-old primipara. The patient had no symptoms. The entire cervix is covered with leukoplakial patches. The right side of the cervix is pictured. White plaques, some of which can be wiped away, are observed over the entire cervix without application of 3% acetic acid. Underneath, fine punctation and mosaic structures are visible between 7 and 8 o'clock.

The histologic assessment supported the colposcopic finding.

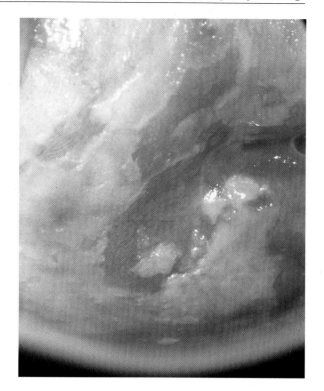

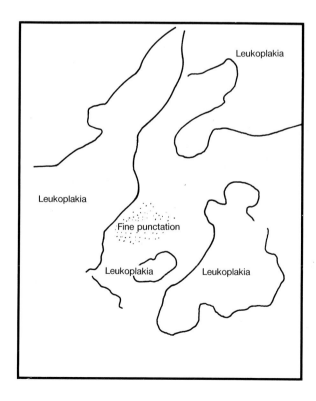

Fig. 4.103: Fine leukoplakia

Patient: 48-year-old para 3. Large, whitish keratotic areas are visible at the anterior as well as posterior cervical os even without the application of 3% acetic acid. The keratotic area is somewhat elevated from the normal epithelial surface. The patient had no symptoms.

Histologic findings: hyperkeratosis.

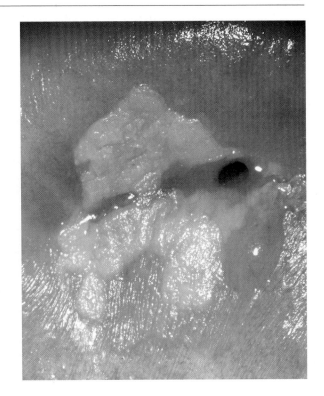

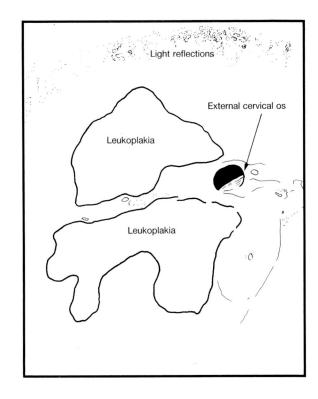

Fig. 4.104: Coarse leuko-plakia

Patient: 20 years old. On the left side of the external os one can see a whitish, patchy thickening of the epithelium that tends to bleed easily. The abnormal epithelium is partly detached from the base. This finding is typical of coarse leukoplakia and should be regarded as highly suspicious of possible malignancy. Histologic examination is mandatory, even if the cytologic (Papanicolaou) smear is negative. This patient unfortunately failed to return for further evaluation.

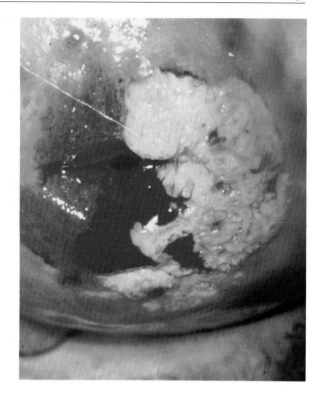

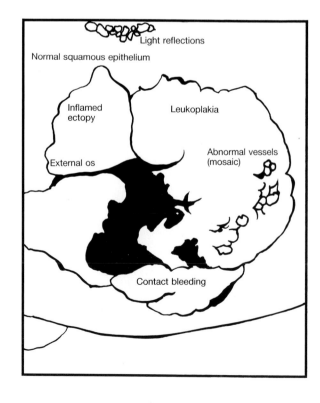

Fig. 4.105: Coarse leuko-plakia

Patient: 44-year-old gravida 2. The cervical surface is covered with numerous patches of coarse leukoplakia. These are easily recognized as thick, whitish, elevated areas even prior to the use of acetic acid. Such a finding must be histologically assessed. The cervical (Papanicolaou) smear is IV in this case.

Histologic findings: carcinoma in situ – CIN III.

The patient has not had a gynecologic examination in 14 years.

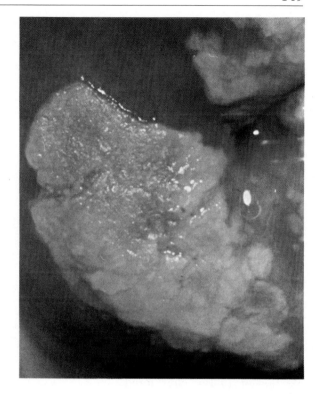

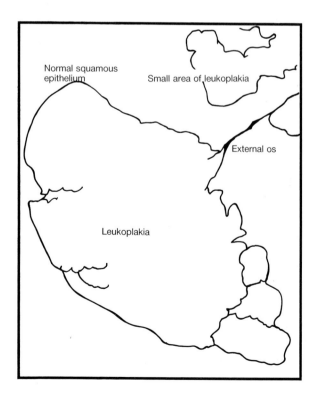

Normal squamous epithelium

Small area of leukoplakia

External os

Leukoplakia

**Fig. 4.106: Coarse leuko-
plakia (Compare with
Fig. 4.105)**

Patient: 27 years old. The
situation is similar to that in
Fig. 4.105. The Papanicolaou
smear was IV. Elevated scaly
white epithelial areas are visible at the cervical os without
the application of 3% acetic
acid. These areas can be
wiped away in some spots.
Between 6 and 7 o'clock one
can also recognize coarse, irregular mosaic structures.

A large nabothian cyst with
markedly branching vessels
was also found.

Histologic findings (conization): severe dysplasia on
the border to the carcinoma
in situ – CIN III.

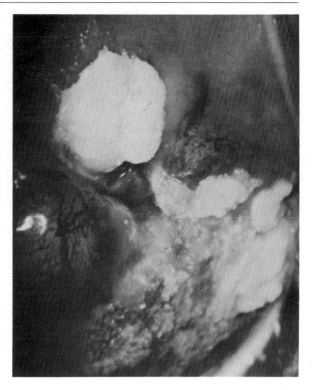

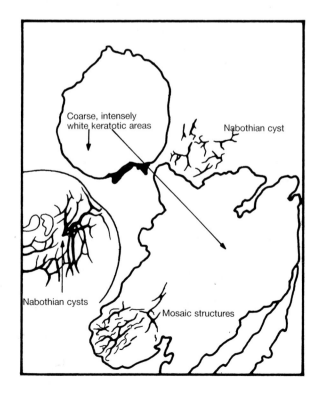

4.3.5 Atypical Transformation Zone/ White Epithelium

The difficulty in classifying and interpreting atypical colposcopic findings has been repeatedly emphasized. This holds true especially for the atypical transformation zone, which challenges the colposcopist again and again. The incidence according to several authors is between 0.2% and 3%.

COUPEZ, CARRERA, and DEXEUS differentiate between an atypical reepithelization with the formation of a stable atypical scar, ie, a metaplastic process, and a true atypical transformation zone. The latter goes through three phases during its development:

1. Areas of punctation, mosaic, and – after application of acetic acid – whitish squamous epithelium appear at the outer edges of the ectopy.
2. Starting at the periphery, the ectopy tends to disappear progressively, leaving only the grapelike structures of the columnar epithelium visible at the center. At this stage, mainly whitish squamous epithelium (after use of acetic acid) can be recognized next to peculiar gland openings surrounded by a circular rim.
3. In the third phase, the entire columnar epithelium has disappeared. The reepithelization has been completed, leaving only whitish epithelium after application of acetic acid and, for example, areas of mosaic and punctation.

These authors classify this type of lesion as benign but later mention that carcinoma in situ can be found in 0.43% and severe dysplasia in 0.86% on histologic examination. This indicates that one cannot speak of a benign metaplastic change. The true atypical transformation zone is thereby severely limited. Notwithstanding, the authors point out how extremely difficult it is to furnish a clear definition. The following colposcopic findings are described as parameters for the atypical transformation zone:

Red, bleeding or erosive areas, frequently found at the periphery
Macerated foci giving a very significant indication of atypia
Gland openings with white keratotic rims, opalescent or whitish epithelium with red patches, and whitish borders occurring in varying proportions and irregular shapes.

Not infrequently, these alterations can be recognized without using acetic acid. Their outline is ill defined and blurred. Columnar ectopy can be found centrally in exceptional cases. The vascularization pattern is commonly irregular. Mosaic, punctation, and leukoplakia may occur.

Instead of "atypical transformation zone" MESTWERDT and WESPI use the term *unusual transformation zone,* which they describe as:

Marked increase of vessel formation
Easily bleeding epithelial defects
Hyperemia mostly due to infection
Irregular surface contour of the transformation zone and damlike elevation at the border.

COPPLESON, PIXLEY, and REID divide the atypical transformation zone into three grades:

1. Smooth white epithelium with or without regular vessels of fine caliber
2. Smooth, even whiter epithelium with or without irregular vessels of large caliber
3. Very white epithelium with coiled vessels of large caliber giving the appearance of papillary epithelium owing to irregular surface contour.

STAFL and KOLSTAD use the term atypical transformation zone only in connection with leukoplakia, basketlike lesions, punctation, mosaic, and atypical vascularization. They state that the whitish color of the squamous epithelium resembles leukoplakia, except for the absence of visible terminal vessels. The main differences from true leukoplakia are that these changes can be seen only after application of acetic acid and that they are level with the surrounding epithelium. From all of these different interpretations of the atypical transformation zone one can see how controversial the subject is. The ambiguity of this lesion complex — that is, the difficulty of differentiating between typical and atypical transformation zone — has persisted over the years. This is repeatedly stressed in German literature. Personally, I have consistently emphasized that the vascularized areas demand special attention. The basic criterion for all forms of transformation zone is the (acetic) white epithelium: The longer the white discoloration remains after acetic acid application, and the more intensive the stain, the more suspicious the findings. The marked vascularization within the transformation zone has always been — and remains — very much a problem! Atypical vessels are known to occur when an inflammatory process is involved — and inflammation is frequently present in patients presenting for evaluation. To simplify diagnosis, especially for the beginning colposcopist, in transformation zone, I present an attempt at systematic classification (Table 4.1).

This classification system, like all others, suffers from the defect of being incomplete, and obviously there are smooth transitions!

Grade I atypical transformation zone is characterized by changes described under points 1 and 2 (without a or b). The white epithelium is fine and is level with the surrounding mucosa. No major vascular changes occur.

Table 4.1 *Colposcopic Criteria for Diagnosis of Atypical Transformation Zone*

1. *Squamous epithelium that turns white after application of 3% acetic acid* (in contrast to leukoplakia); the more intensely the epithelium stains and the longer the discoloration holds, the more suspicious the findings
2. Within the white epithelium there are *gland openings* with a red base and frequently a whitish keratotic rim or a vascular red margin; these gland openings may present with either
   a. a nichelike depression (hardly to be differentiated from "nichelike *Felderung*" [see 4.3.2] or
   b. a papillary protuberance (like the fingertip of a glove)
3. *Erosions*
4. All forms of *atypical vascularization:* mosaic, punctation, hairpin capillaries, corkscrew capillaries, disturbed intercapillary intervals, bizarre and broken-off vessels of varied caliber
5. Leukoplakia
6. Irregular surface contour
7. Fragility

Grade II atypical transformation zone involves changes in groups 1, 2, 3, and 4, with possibly a slight irregularity in surface contour.

Grade III atypical transformation zone is characterized foremost by an irregular surface level and fragility. The white epithelium is intensely colored and the effect is longlasting. All criteria points (1–7) are observed.

When attempting to diagnose histologic atypia on the basis of colposcopic findings, the following should be considered:

Grade I atypical transformation zone requires only observation. Of course, a cytologic smear is also made. Histologically, an "abnormal" or "simple atypical" epithelium as defined by HINSELMANN is found in such cases.

Grade II atypical transformation zone histologically shows a mild to moderate dysplasia (CIN I–III).

Usually, in grade III atypical transformation zone, histologic examination reveals an existing carcinoma in situ (CIN III) or a developing carcinoma.

The more experienced the examiner, the more easily an atypical transformation zone is classified. When a grade II atypical transformation zone is diagnosed, one should be generous with taking biopsies, in particular, when the cytologic smear is negative.

An interpretation of the malignancy is extremely difficult. Individual authors give such varying accounts that a comparison is problematic. The preceding text describes the problems involved in interpretation when classifying atypical transformation zones.

The incidence of malignancy was found by LIMBURG to be 7.8%, whereas BAJARDI reports it to be 17% and COUPEZ and associates as high as 54%.

Fig. 4.107: Grade I atypical transformation zone

Patient: 37 years old. The most important criterion of an atypical transformation zone is visible at the posterior cervical lip: squamous epithelium that turns white after the use of acetic acid. This lesion has tonguelike extensions between 5 and 7 o'clock in a posterior direction. There are also numerous gland openings, which appear like punched-out holes with a red base and some with a keratinized rim. A fine mosaic can be seen on the anterior cervical lip close to the external os.

The slightly atypical epithelium of this 37-year-old patient was observed to be unchanged for 10 years. Repeat cytologic (Papanicolaou) smears proved negative.

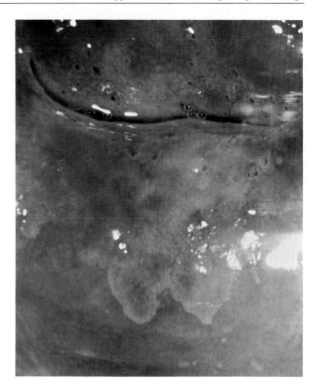

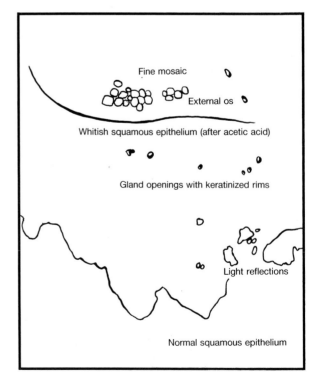

Fine mosaic

External os

Whitish squamous epithelium (after acetic acid)

Gland openings with keratinized rims

Light reflections

Normal squamous epithelium

Fig. 4.108: Grade I atypical transformation zone

Patient: 36-year-old para 2 with recurring vaginal discharge. A fine white epithelial area with mosaic structures at the anterior cervical lip. Ectopic islands and gland openings with keratotic rims are also observed. The colpophotograph shows a section of the anterior cervical lip.

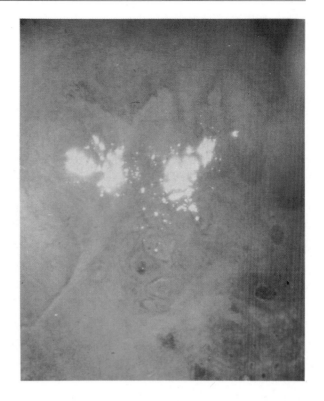

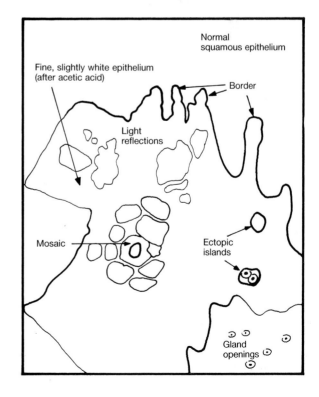

Fig. 4.109: Grade I atypical transformation zone

This 19-year-old, who had been taking oral contraceptives for 2 years, presented with a central polypoid ectopy undergoing metaplasia. The tissue shows a certain vulnerability, and there are areas of fine white epithelium (after acetic acid) bordering the normal epithelium, also fine punctation and mosaic.

A severe inflammation is present, which makes the colposcopic finding difficult to interpret in regard to atypia.

The histologic examination of a punch biopsy showed a severely inflamed ectopy with advanced metaplasia by squamous epithelium, which had also grown into the apertures of the mucosal crypts. The Papanicolaou smear was classified IV. In addition, a severe adnexitis with a high blood sedimentation rate was found.

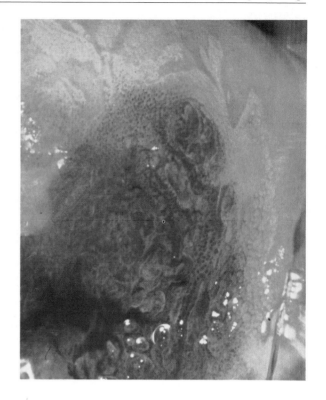

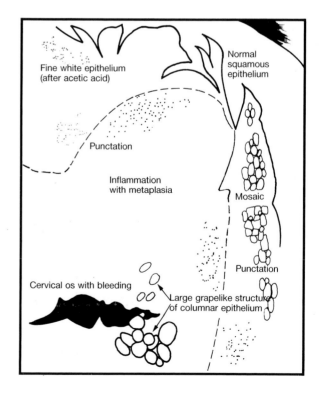

Fig. 4.110: Grade II atypical transformation zone

Patient: 35-year-old para 3. The posterior cervical lip shows an area of erosion with bleeding tendency at about 6 o'clock. This lesion comprises a genuine epithelial defect. Another criterion demonstrating the atypical transformation zone is the presence of whitish squamous epithelium after application of acetic acid. Many gland openings with a red base and white keratotic rim can be seen, some of them having a papillary appearance.

If several parameters indicate the transformation zone to be atypical – as in this case – histologic evaluation should be carried out even if the cytologic (Papanicolaou) smear is negative. A colposcopically directed punch biopsy was performed.

Histologic findings: mild dysplasia – CIN I.

The patient returned for regular colposcopic and cytologic monitoring, which indicated an almost complete regression of the atypical epithelial changes.

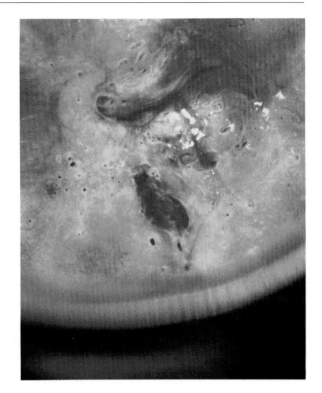

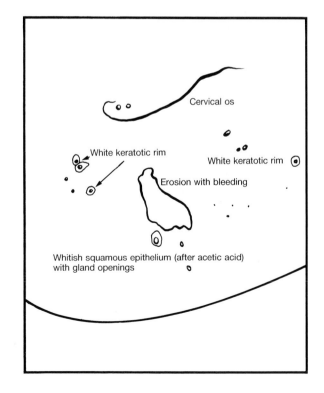

Cervical os

White keratotic rim

White keratotic rim

Erosion with bleeding

Whitish squamous epithelium (after acetic acid) with gland openings

Fig. 4.111: Grade II atypical transformation zone

Patient: 33-year-old primi-para. The anterior cervical lip shows epithelium turned white upon application of acetic acid, with cavity-like gland openings. Irregular mosaic and individual puncta-tion are found at about 1 o'clock. The observed changes are to a certain extent coarse, that is, they clearly protrude from the normal epithelial sur-face level. The cytologic (Papanicolaou) smear was III. Histologic findings (cone biop-sy): moderate dysplasia – CIN II.

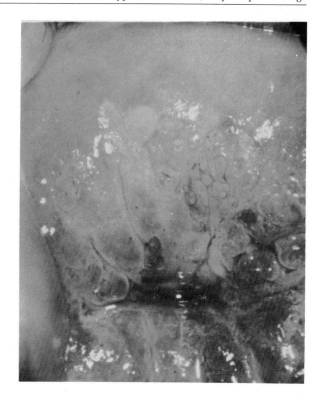

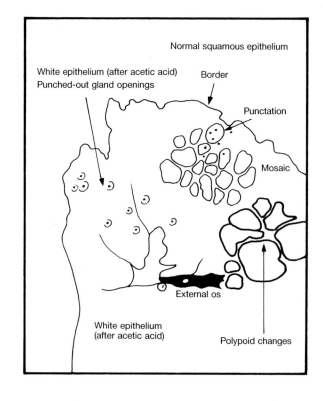

Fig. 4.112: Grade II atypical transformation zone

Patient: 36-year-old para I with history of oral contraceptive use. The criteria of atypical transformation zone are especially pronounced on the anterior cervical lip. The tissue vulnerability has led to small, slightly bleeding erosions. In addition, irregular mosaic structures and some coarse punctation can be seen in the white-stained epithelium (upon application of acetic acid).

The cytologic (Papanicolaou) smear is III d. The histologic finding after conization is moderate dysplasia – CIN II.

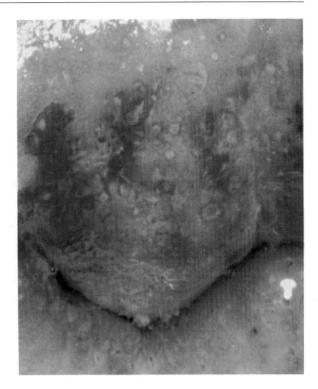

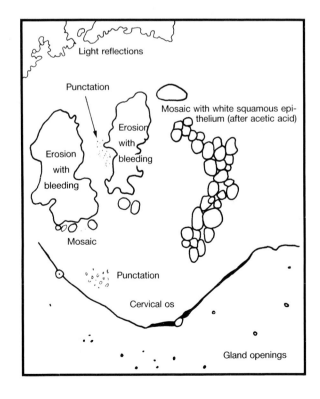

Fig. 4.113: Grade III highly suspicious atypical transformation zone

Patient: 32 years old. The more criteria of an atypical transformation zone are observed, the higher the suspicion of cancer.

In this patient, white squamous epithelium becomes visible, although only slightly stained, at the anterior cervical lip after application of acetic acid. Within this area one can identify red-based and white-rimmed gland openings which, in part, have a papillomatous appearance, protruding like the fingers of a glove. Atypical vascularization with a mosaic and punctation pattern is visible between 11 and 1 o'clock. White squamous epithelium is also present on the posterior cervical lip.

A very thorough colposcopic examination is necessary because the most important criterion of atypical changes is the protruding gland openings, which are very difficult to recognize.

The other atypical changes are only minimally developed. The cytologic (Papanicolaou) smear is IV.

Histologic findings (vaginal hysterectomy): severe dysplasia – CIN III.

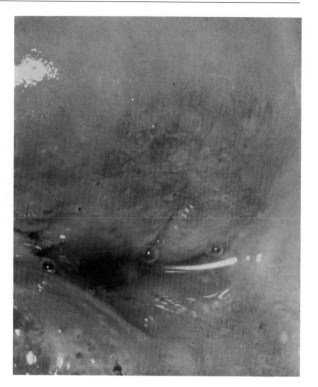

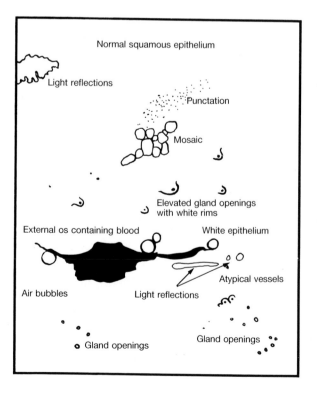

Fig. 4.114: Highly suspicious grade III atypical transformation zone

Patient: 46-year-old para 2 who had not been examined gynecologically for 9 years. The posterior cervical lip shows coarse punctation mainly between 5 and 7 o'clock. Note the increased intercapillary distance as seen at 4 o'clock. Coarse punctation is also seen toward the posterior cervical lip. Further, extreme tissue vulnerability has led to small bleeding erosions. Close to the external os one can see the white epithelium (after acetic acid) particularly well; large gland openings have a punched-out appearance, a whitish rim, and a red base. There is a fairly distinct border to the normal squamous epithelium.

Cytologic findings: Papanicolaou IV a.

Histologic findings: carcinoma in situ – CIN III.

Therapy: vaginal hysterectomy.

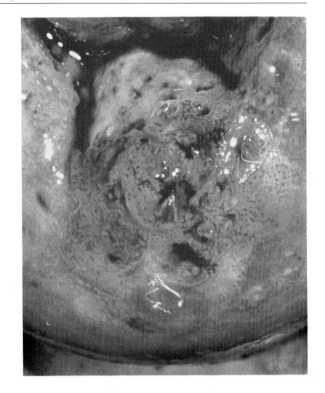

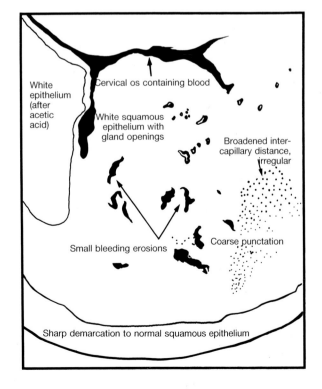

Fig. 4.115: Grade III atypical transformation zone

Patient: 31-year-old primipara. Coarse, distinctly white area (after application of acetic acid) at the posterior cervical lip with irregular punctation and obvious differences in surface level. The atypical epithelial area extends to the cervical canal; irregular mosaic is observed around 11 o'clock and coarse punctation at 1 o'clock.

Cytologic findings: Papanicolaou smear is IV a.

Histologic findings (conization): carcinoma in situ CIN III.

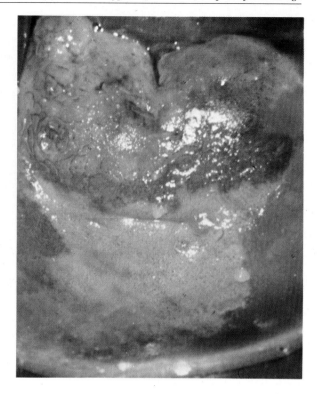

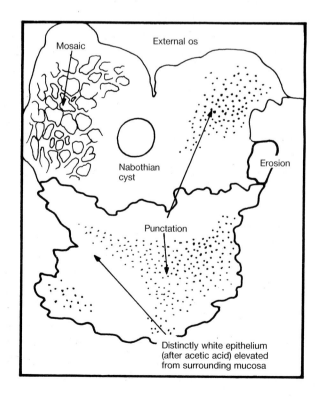

4.3.6 Papilloma/condyloma

The international nomenclature still classifies papillomas and condylomas under "various colposcopic findings." In recent years, however, an increased number of histologic atypias have been diagnosed among papillomatous changes, ranging from mild dysplasia – CIN I to carcinoma in situ – CIN III. The identification of papillomatous tumors, especially when these are vulnerable and show vascular atypia, may signify an already clinically manifest carcinoma (See section 4.3.7).

To distinguish colposcopically between condyloma and papilloma can be very difficult, but certain differentiations can be made. Condylomas have a more wart-like appearance with patchy, elevated protrusions and very typical papillary development that often has a fine, tuftlike appearance. Condylomas are usually a multiple occurrence. Papillomas, on the other hand, generally occur singly and stain white upon application of acetic acid. They often show a papillomatous, villous-type surface structure. Such changes are found at the cervix, vagina, and vulva.

According to HAMPERL, these histologically benign lesions belong to the group of fibroepithelial tumors that derive from surface areas where the integument consists of squamous epithelium, as found in the lower female genital tract. HAMPERL describes the histopathologic tissue composition of these tumors as follows: The covering squamous epithelium is thickened, with interspersed elongated stromal papillae that separate the epithelium into massive blocks. The tumor protrudes in patchlike fashion. Another possibility is retraction of the epithelium between the papillae, causing an uneven surface with fine tufts or buds. Finally, the stromal papillae, while merging toward the surface, can form small lateral secondary projections, leading to either fine or somewhat bulky proliferations with rounded or pointed endings. The tumor then has a cauliflower-like appearance which may be seen colposcopically. The villi may be narrow or more plump. The villi often contain blood vessels and present colposcopically as atypical vascularization like that seen in punctation. Visible are corkscrew capillaries, comma-shaped, or broken-off capillaries, and more.

An important criterion for differentiation, according to MADEJ, is the following: If the atypical vessels disappear after application of acetic acid (this author uses 5% lactic acid) – or, in other words, if only distinctly white-stained epithelium is seen with villi formation – the papilloma can be considered benign. If the vascular structure remains, however, then the lesion is most likely a premalignant alteration. An important differentiating criterion here too is: If the epithelium stains intensely white and holds the color over a long period, this is also an indication of histologic atypia for condyloma/papilloma.

The etiology of condylomas or papillomas has long been known to be infectious, usually by means of a virus.

Scientific research, in particular by the ZUR HANSEN, GISSMANN and DURST group, has identified a number of papilloma virus types in recent years. Today we know that HPV 16 and HPV 18 are found more often in carcinoma and its preliminary stages. Herpesvirus 16 is found in approximately 50% of cervical carcinoma and in about 40% of carcinoma in situ – CIN III, and in as many as 80% of cases of carcinoma in situ of the vulva = Morbus Bowen. Hyperviruses 6 and 11 are usually found in condyloma acuminatum. These are benign changes.

As has already been mentioned, the incidence of viral diseases of the female genital tract has increased greatly in recent years. MEISELS pointed out the cytologic significance of condylomas caused by viral infections in 1976 and 1981. Changes of this sort are seen most often in women under 30. However, no causal relationship between virus and carcinomatous development has been proved to date. ZUR HANSEN mentions the reciprocal action between specific papilloma virus infections and chemical or physical carcinogenic agents in cells. Viral DNA is always present in the cell.

To summarize: So far, no causal relationship between viral infection and carcinogenesis has been proved. Without a doubt, however, both papilloma virus type 16 and papilloma virus type 18 are risk factors. Often, inflammation with vaginal discharge is found in the presence of condyloma/papilloma. A number of bacteria, fungi, and spirilla can be detected. Inflammation can make interpretation of colposcipic findings especially difficult. I have already mentioned that the formation of atypical vascularization can be frequently seen at the tips of stromal papillae.

Histologic assessment is required in these cases even if the cytologic (Papanicolaou) smear is negative. Here again, the rule is: better to do one histologic examination too many than one too few!

The cases I have observed so far involved a range of conditions from dysplasia through to carcinoma in situ (CIN I–III). Such cases are also described in the literature. The papillary surface often appears shiny and whitish – pearl-like. Marked keratinization is often present, in which case no vessels are visible. To me it seems especially important to use colposcopic examination to differentiate between the smooth and the papillomatous forms of condylomas. A criteria for histologic evaluation are: if (1) the *smooth condyloma* stains intensely white and remains stained, and if (2) coarse, irregular mosaic or punctation is observed, then taking a biopsy is essential. The significance of fine, slightly white-stained areas, at the mucosal level usually with fine punctation and/or mosaic structures, should not be exaggerated; it suffices to note their presence. I have followed up on such minor abnormal changes for as long as 20 years, and not one case showed premalignant or malignant development. Special attention should be paid to the already mentioned *atypical papilloma,* with its very distinct vascular atypias. The atypical vessels generally remain visible even after the application of 3% acetic acid solution, in contrast to benign changes in which the vessels disappear.

Finally, mention must be made of the so-called *verrucae vulgaris,* which are classified with viral infections. The herpes infections HPV types 1 and 2 also belong in this group. In the United States, dermatologic studies have shown that genital herpes is the second most common sexually transmitted disease (after gonorrhea). Examples are presented in Figs. 4.47 and 4.48.

So long as the so-called hybrid method is used, viral identification is not possible, and it is very difficult in practice to prove viral origin with certainty. If the cytologic smear shows koilocytes and keratotic cells, the presence of a viral infection is assumed. In the meantime, additional virus types have been identified, for example, HPV 31, 33, 35, 39, 41, and 43. To date we know that types 33 and 35 have been found in cervical carcinoma and its prestages.

Fig. 4.116: Papilloma

Patient: 19-year-old with 3-year history of oral contraceptive use. The posterior cervical lip shows a large papillomatous area abundant with atypical vessels (hairpin and corkscrew capillaries, suggestion of mosaic and punctation). These can be observed without the application of 3% acetic acid. After swabbing with acetic acid the atypical vessels disappear, which is generally indicative of a benign process. The papilloma extended into the external os. The cytologic (Papanicolaou) smear was III d.

Histologic findings: condyloma.

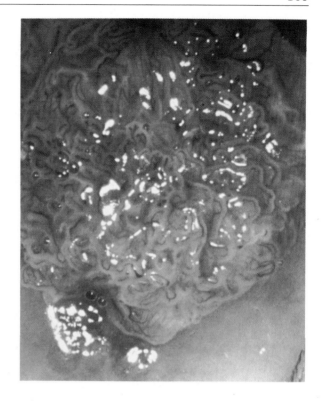

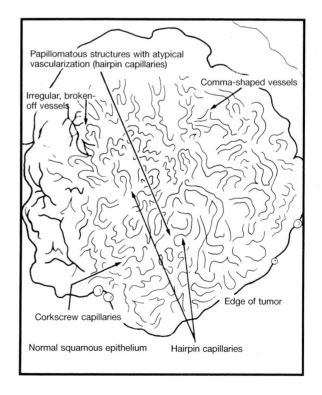

Fig. 4.117: Papilloma

Patient: 24-year-old with 6-year history of oral contraceptive use. A multilobular papillomatous tumor is visible on the edge of a strongly proliferative and unsuspicious ectopy. The upper lobe shows very distinct tongue-shaped papillae in which hairpin capillaries are easily recognizable after the application of acetic acid. The lower lobe presents atypical vessels with a splattered and irregular appearance. Next to the papilloma, between 2 and 4 o'clock, are areas of mosaic and punctation. Even if the cytologic (Papanicolaou) smear is negative, such findings should always be evaluated histologically. This patient failed to return for her follow-up examination.

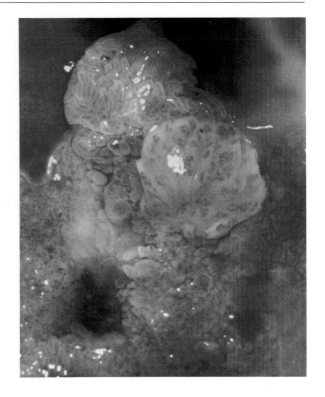

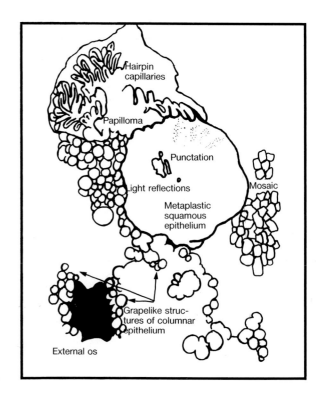

Fig. 4.118: Papilloma

Patient: 24-year-old with IUD in place for 2 years. A papilloma with atypical vessels (punctation) is seen at the anterior cervical lip. Furthermore, a normal transformation zone can be identified. This 24-year-old patient had an intrauterine contreceptive device inserted 2 years ago.

Such a colposcopic finding must always be regarded as suspicious and should have histologic clarification even if the cytologic (Papanicolaou) smear is negative.

The histologic examination of a colposcopically directed punch biopsy showed a columnar ectopy with chronic inflammation being covered by a thick layer of squamous epithelium that partly outlined the cervical crypts.

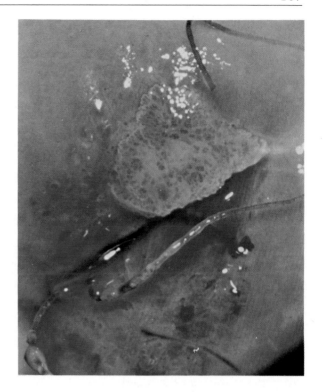

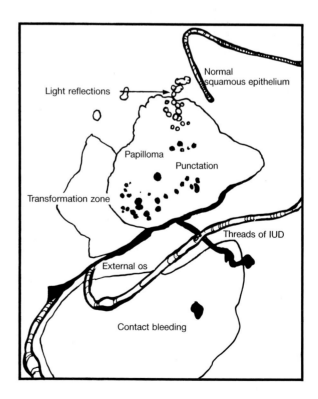

Fig. 4.119: Papilloma

Patient: Asymptomatic 18-year-old nullipara. There is a large papilloma with papillae-like protrusions, in which individual small comma-shaped capillaries are visible at the anterior cervical lip. This observation is possible after the application of 3% acetic acid. A normal ectopy undergoing transformation is seen, principally at the posterior cervical lip. Even prior to acetic acid application, a pronounced white discoloration can be seen here, indicating keratinization.

Histologic findings of a directed biopsy: typical condyloma with severe acanthosis and parakeratosis. There is also some infiltration of squamous epithelium into the gland openings.

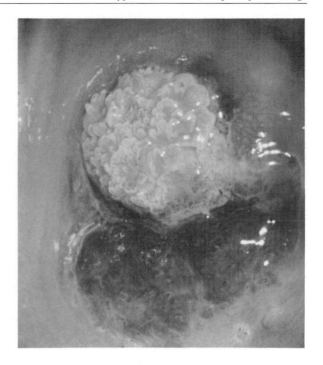

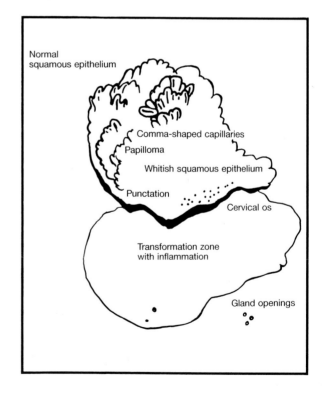

Fig. 4.120: Papilloma with mosaic and punctation

Patient: 22-year-old nullipara. The entire cervical surface is covered by a transformation zone that is partly papillomatous, showing areas of mosaic and punctation at the periphery (the colpophotograph demonstrates a section of the anterior cervical lip). This kind of finding indicates that the squamous epithelium has already undergone a certain degree of keratinization. Still, the lesion is noteworthy enough to require histologic clarification. A cervical conization was performed. The histologic examination showed mild dysplasia – CIN I.

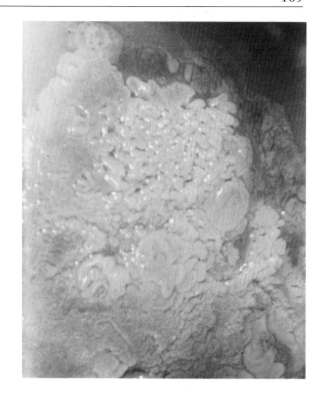

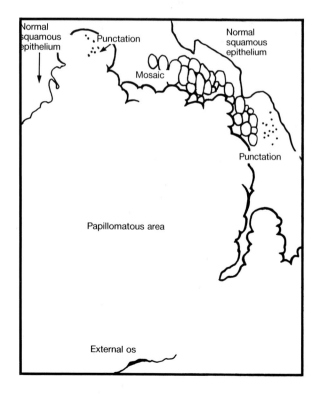

Fig. 4.121: Condyloma

Patient: 23-year-old primipara posthysterectomy. A cherrystone-sized, whitish, wartlike tumor is seen at the vaginal vault. The lesion demonstrates easily recognizable whitish buds on the surface which have punctation-like vessels at their endings. This 23-year-old primipara had previously undergone vaginal hysterectomy to resect a cervical carcinoma in situ. She now reported severe vaginal discharge due to *Candida* infection.

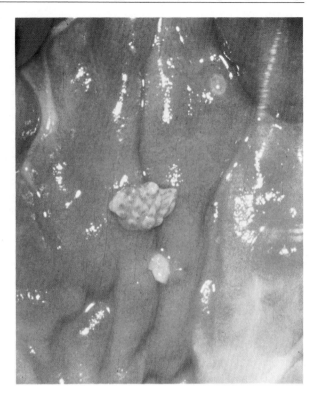

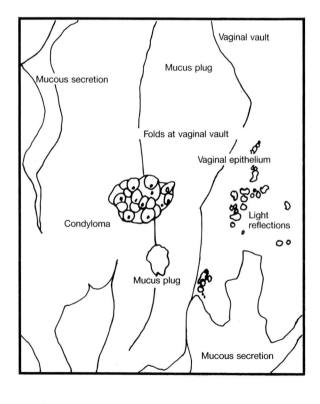

Fig. 4.122: Multiple condylomas in the vagina

Patient: 52-year-old primipara posthysterectomy. This patient had undergone a hysterectomy after a uterine myomatosus had been diagnosed. Inflammation of the vagina and vulva were repeatedly treated. The patient now reported a severe itching sensation around the vagina and pressure on the bladder. Small, pointed condylomas were found throughout the entire vagina. The colpophotograph shows the left vaginal wall. A checkup examination after 6 months showed the two condylomas to have spontaneously disappeared.

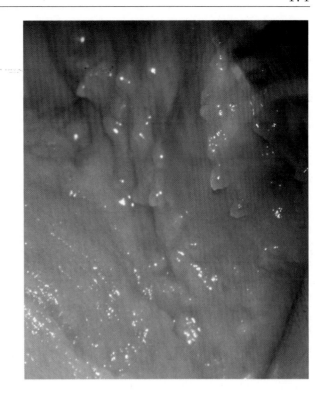

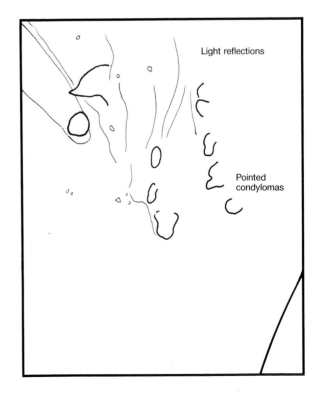

Fig. 4.123: Large papilloma with punctation at the cervical vault

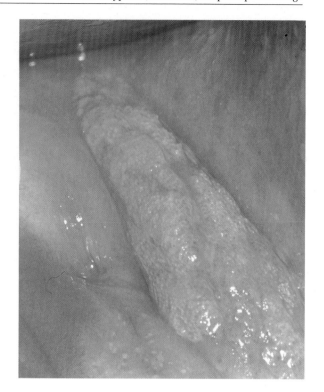

Patient: 43-year-old, 3 years posthysterectomy. On the left side of the vaginal fundus there is a long, protruding, intensely white-stained papillomatous mass with recognizable punctation. After 2 years this process showed total regression.

This case is a particularly impressive argument for the necessity of using both colposcopy and cytology when examining a patient. The patient had undergone abdominal hysterectomy (no suspicion of malignancy) when she was 40. Three years later, when the patient was 43 years old, cytologic (Papanicolaou) smears were made with very serious results: moderate to severe dysplagia, with the possibility of carcinoma in situ not to be ruled out. Repeated smears gave similar results. Histologic assessment was mandatory. The patient was referred to me for conization, since biopsying is routine in such a case. For various reasons (foremost the absolute refusal of the patient), however, I decided on observation. Followup examinations, over a period of 7 years to date, showed completely normal colposcopic as well as cytologic findings.

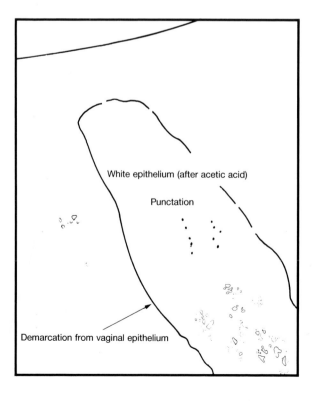

White epithelium (after acetic acid)

Punctation

Demarcation from vaginal epithelium

Fig. 4.124: Smooth condyloma

Patient: 27-year-old nullipara. Small fine white areas are observed upon application of acetic acid in the left corner of the cervical os. Condylomas have also been identified close to the anal ring. Condylomas in this area and in the vulva had already been discovered more than 2 years previously. The patient is therefore undergoing treatment (laser and interferon).

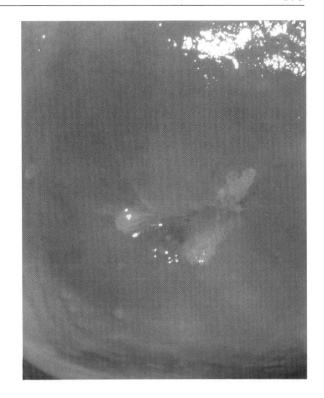

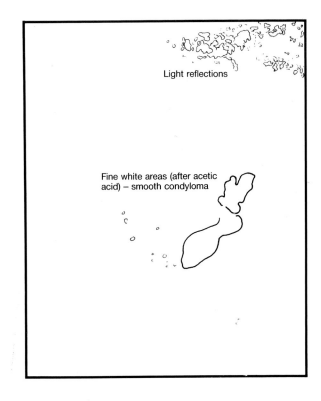

Fig. 4.125: Vulval condyloma

Patient: 21-year-old nullipara. Several large nodules
were observed near the vulva.
The patient presented with severe pruritus and vaginal discharge. Excision was per-
formed with electrocoagulation when the nodules showed
signs of expanding.
Histologic findings: condyloma
acuminatum.

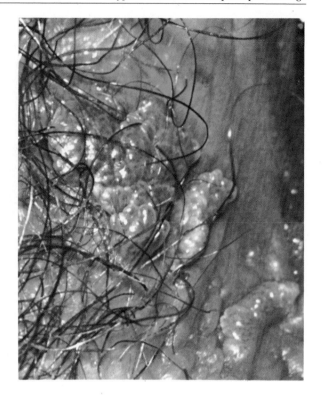

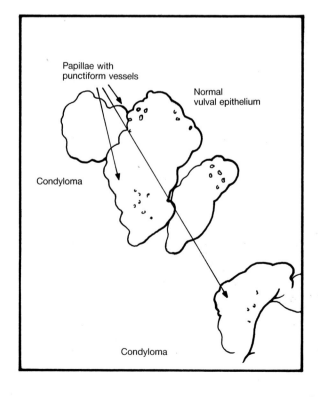

Fig. 4.126: Vulval condyloma

Two large condyloma-like structures are found near the vulva. The condyloma lying more proximal has the typical villous-shaped form, while the more distal condyloma is dark-bluish. The surface has a broad villous and rather plump appearance. Blood vessels are not visible.

Histologic findings: condyloma.

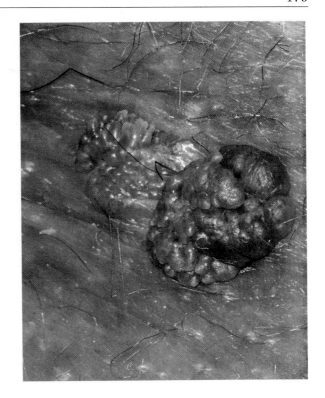

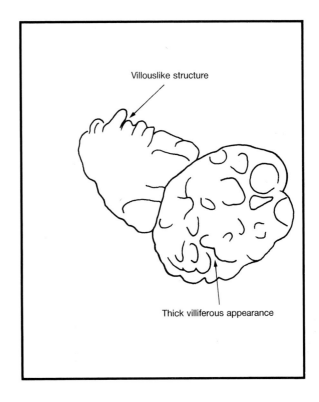

Villouslike structure

Thick villiferous appearance

Fig. 4.127: Large vulval papilloma

Patient: 73 years old. A large, multilobular, whitish tumor is found near the right vulval lip; the surface shows a papillomatous structure. The patient presented with no symptoms.

Histologic findings: papilloma.

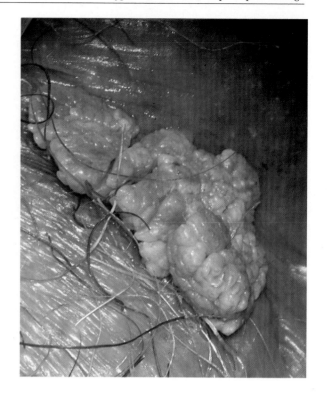

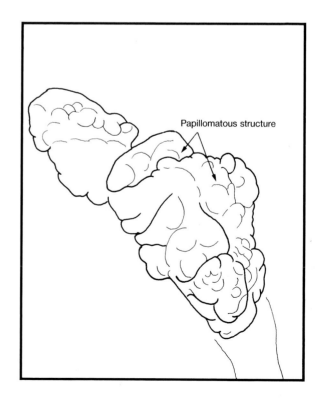

Papillomatous structure

Fig. 4.128: Cervical condyloma (See also Fig. 4.129)

This 25-year-old patient presented with recurring vaginal discharge. One recognizes three circular, slightly elevated condylomatous areas on the anterior cervical lip.
Histologic findings: condyloma with mild to moderate dysplasia – CIN I to II.

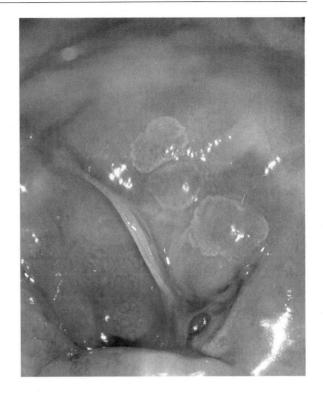

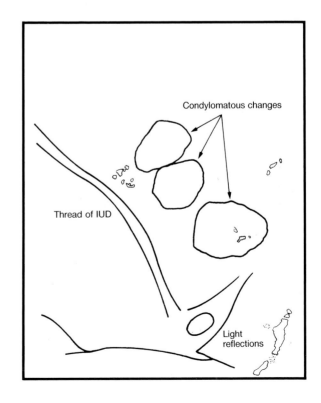

Fig. 4.129: Atypical cervical condyloma (See also Fig. 4.128)

Patient: same as in Fig. 4.128 three years later. A large papillomatous area with splotchy, coarse punctation is seen on the posterior cervical lip. On the anterior cervical lip one also recognizes white epithelium (after applying acetic acid) and an indication of mosaic structure. In addition, condylomatous changes are also seen near the right corner of the cervical os. Although the cytologic (Papanicolaou) smear had been negative so far, it is now IV.

Histologic assessment (conization): condyloma and ca in situ = CIN III.

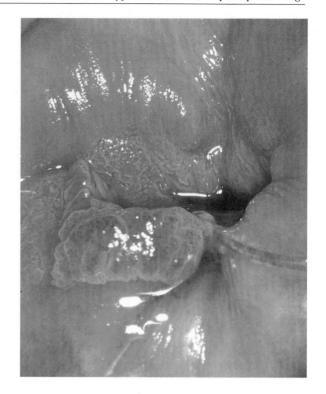

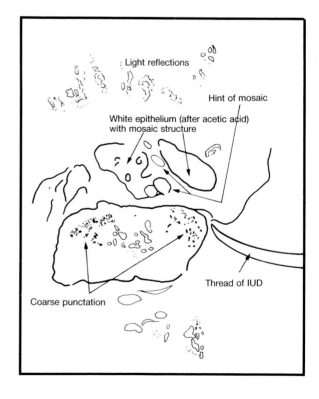

4.3.7 Findings Suspicious of Carcinoma (Atypical Vascularization/ Exophytic Changes/Ulcer)

Colposcopic findings in cases of early carcinoma – mainly group Ia microcarcinomas and group Ib cervical carcinomas – are typically characterized principally by atypical vascularization. Their pattern can be diverse, presenting as coarse mosaic or punctation, bizarrely shaped and broken-off vessels, corkscrew arteries, and hairpin capillaries. Of great importance are the variations in caliber and the increased intercapillary distance. An adaptive vascular hypertrophy is often visible at the elevated rimlike border of more advanced cancers.

For inspection of the blood vessels, it is recommended that the green filter be interposed and that 3% acetic acid be used. An ordinary colposcope with 10× to 15× magnification is insufficient to identify finer detail in the vasculature, although this magnification is adequate for routine practice. Here, higher magnifications have proved valuable. For colposcopic documentation, fine atypical vascular changes are much better evaluated with stereo slides. In addition to atypical vascularization, irregularities in the surface contour and the appearance of bullous, edematous areas within atypical epithelial regions are also indicative of malignant neoplastic growth. If these changes appear bullous and yellowish they are considered exophytic; endophytic growth also occurs. Ulceration – often with an elevated rim – and the previously described adaptive vascular hypertrophy are, however, the predominant features.

The more advanced the carcinogenesis, the less detail is visible through the colposcope. Carcinomatous tissue is usually fragile and bleeds easily when damaged by even minimal swabbing pressure. Bleeding may impede colposcopic assessment; for that reason most cases of advanced carcinoma can be more readily diagnosed by macroscopic inspection than by colposcopy or cytology.

When malignancy is suspected the use of Chrobak's test can be very helpful. The test is positive if the tip of a metal sound easily breaks through the surface owing to the fragility of the carcinomatous tissue. Under such conditions one can usually obtain a small specimen of the tissue without difficulty in order to confirm the diagnosis histologically.

**Fig. 4.130: Suspected car-
cinoma – coarse punctation,
severe atypical vascularization (See also Fig. 4.131)**

Patient: 46-year-old nullipara. The patient presented
for a routine examination. The
use of oral contraceptives had
caused no symptoms. After
application of 3% acetic acid, a
distinctly extended epithelial
area became visible near the
anterior cervical lip; the
epithelium stained only slightly white. Numerous gland
openings are visible. Severe
atypical vascularization is
evident between 11 and 4
o'clock: coarse punctation,
coarse mosaic, broken-off irregular capillaries, and tubu-
lar capillaries are in abund-
ance. Severe tissue vulnerability led to small bleeding erosions. This finding is very suspicious of a severe atypia.
Histologic findings: aside from
carcinoma in situ – CIN III, a
microcarcinoma was found
between 2 and 4 o'clock
(where the atypical vascularization is most evident), depth
of growth 2 mm.
Cytologic finding: Papanicolaou IVa – IVb (suspicion of
invasion)
Therapy: hysterectomy.

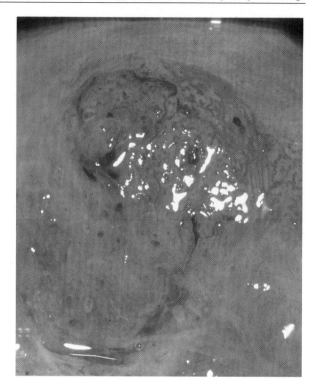

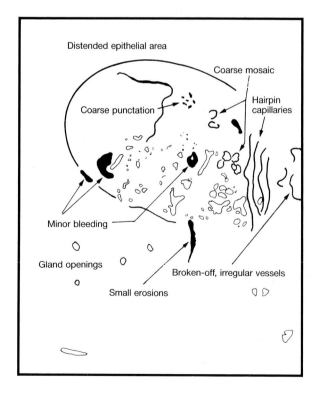

Fig. 4.131: Suspected carcinoma – coarse punctation, severe atypical vascularization (See also Fig. 4.130)

Patient: same as in Fig. 4.130. Note difference after insertion of a green filter. Coarse punctation and coarse irregular mosaic structures as well as broken-off and completely irregular vessels appear much more distinct. Also clearly recognizable are the differences in surface level within the atypical epithelial area and a slightly bullous, damlike rim near the external os. Severe tissue vulnerability indicates a tendency toward bleeding. The atypical epithelial area has already taken on a crater-like appearance in part as seen in clinical carcinoma.

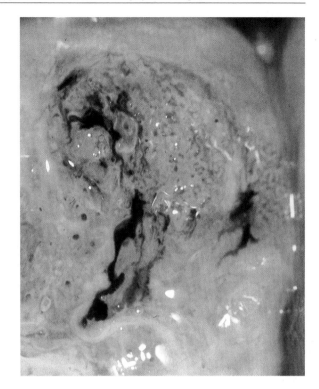

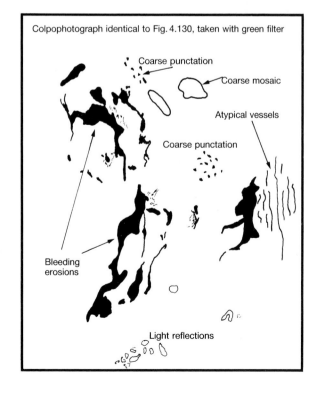

Colpophotograph identical to Fig. 4.130, taken with green filter

Coarse punctation

Coarse mosaic

Atypical vessels

Coarse punctation

Bleeding erosions

Light reflections

**Fig. 4.132: Suspected car-
cinoma – ulcer, vascular
adaptive hypertrophy**

Patient: 89-year-old para 3.
An ulcer is located near the
vaginal wall. The base of the
ulcer has a slightly lardlike
appearance and raised area in
which atypical vessels are visible, similar to vascular adaptive hypertrophy (according to
HINSELMANN). Histologic confirmation was not possible because the patient died. She
presented with total prolapse
and severe urinary inconti-
nence. A ring pessary had
been in place for over
10 years.

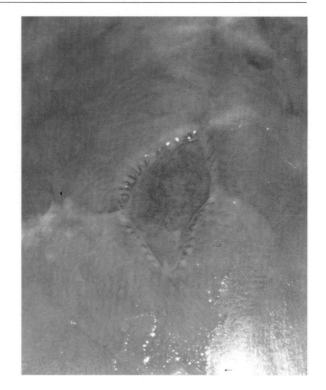

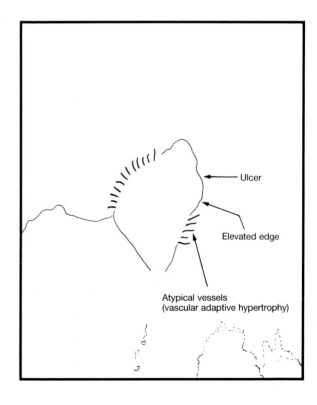

Fig. 4.133: Well demarcated, easily bleeding ulcer on the anterior cervical lip; suspected carcinoma

The edges of the ulcer are slightly elevated. Although atypical vessels are present in the right upper portion, they cannot be clearly seen in this photograph. The base of the ulcer has a punched-out appearance. Such a finding, despite a negative cytologic (Papanicolaou) smear, always requires histologic examination.

Minimal hemorrhage occurred at the cervical os during taking of the cervical smear, which turned out to be negative (Papanicolaou II). This smear was taken from the external os as a routine procedure. The ulcer also has a tendency to bleed.

Histologic findings: microinvasive carcinoma of the cervix.

This case demonstrates how important it is to combine colposcopy with cytology.

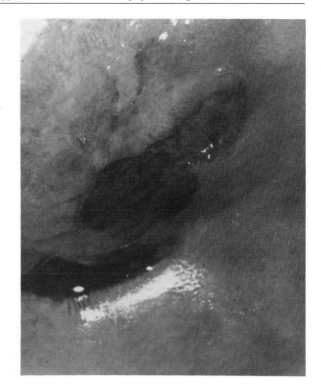

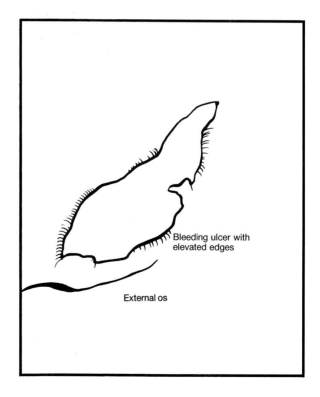

Bleeding ulcer with elevated edges

External os

Fig. 4.134: Papillomatous tumor, suspicion of carcinoma.

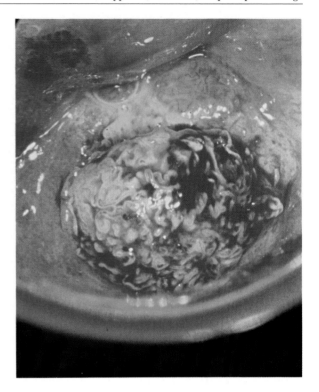

Patient: 50-year-old para 2. A nodular tumor the size of a small cherry is visible on the posterior cervical lip. On the surface of this lesion one can recognize small bleeding erosions and an atypical vascularization pattern (irregular and broken-off vessels and hairpin capillaries). The tumor measures approximately 10 mm wide and 6 mm long. The exact size of the tumor is determined by reading the scale on a film marker that is developed with the negative (1 mm between points). The tumor is surrounded by squamous epithelium which turns white after the use of acetic acid and shows atypical vessels. The bleeding tendency and the marked friability of the tissue with a positive Chrobak test indicate possible malignancy.

Histologic finding: carcinoma. Cytologic finding: Papanicolaou smear, positive V.

Three years ago the patient had a cervical biopsy taken at an outside clinic. Histologically, epithelium with mild atypia was found and the patient underwent electroconization. At the histologic examination of the removed cone specimen no adequate diagnosis was possible because of the tissue damage caused by electrocoagulation. *If atypical epithelium is found on punch biopsy, subsequent conization of the cervix should always be performed with a sharp knife for histologic reevaluation.*

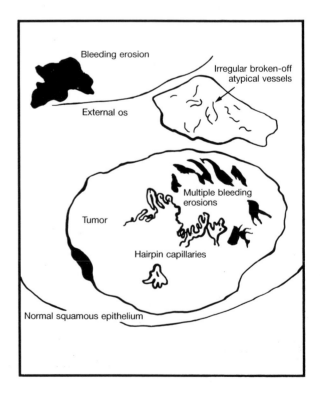

Fig. 4.135: Cervical carcinoma Ib

Patient: 50 years old, one delivery, four spontaneous abortions. The cervix shows ulcerative crater formation with numerous atypical blood vessels. Further important criteria indicating malignancy are the bleeding tendency and the friability of the tissue. The edge of the crater appears elevated and typically demonstrates adaptive vascular hypertrophy. The course of the vessels is irregular, and varying calibers can be identified. This type of finding is already suggestive of carcinoma on macroscopic inspection. Management consisted of a Wertheim-Meigs hysterectomy and postoperative radiotherapy.

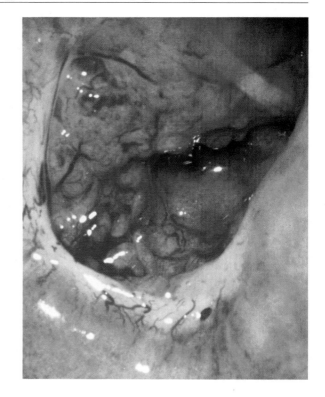

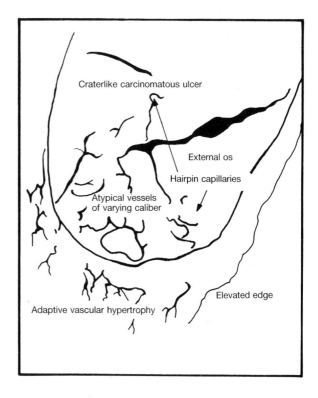

Craterlike carcinomatous ulcer

External os

Hairpin capillaries

Atypical vessels of varying caliber

Elevated edge

Adaptive vascular hypertrophy

Fig. 4.136: Cervical carcinoma III (See also Fig. 4.137)

Patient: 48-year-old gravida 2. At the site of the cervix, a large ulcerative crater has formed. The tissue is extremely friable, and when Chrobak's test was performed, the metal sound easily broke through the surface. There is also a marked bleeding tendency. The actual carcinomatous crater is occupied by a polypoid tissue structure covered by smooth squamous epithelium. Here, too, the Chrobak test is positive. The inexperienced colposcopist might be misled by the smooth appearance of the sqamous epithelium covering the lesion. Figure 4.137 demonstrates the underlying carcinomatous ulcer after removal of the polypoid tissue formation.

The patient reported irregular bleeding for only the past year. Her lower abdominal discomfort and backache could also have been caused by a uterovaginal prolapse that was concurrently present. No gynecologic examination had been performed for years!

Histologically an invasive keratinizing squamous cell carcinoma was found.

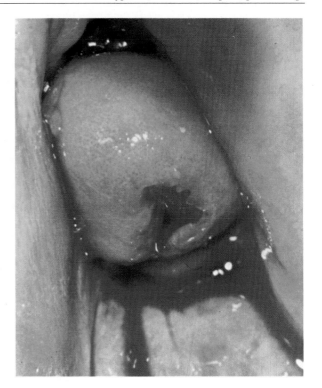

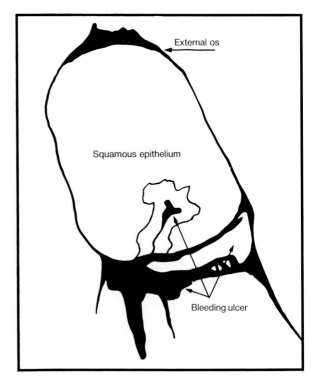

Fig. 4.137: Cervical carcinoma III (See also Fig. 4.136)

Patient: same as in Fig. 4.136. This colpophotograph shows a large, actively bleeding carcinomatous crater after removal of the polypoid structure. The tissue has a papillomatous appearance with atypical vessels. Details are hardly identifiable because of severe bleeding.

As mentioned before, the changes in advanced cervical carcinoma are easier seen macroscopically than through the colposcope.

Because of the superficial tumor necrosis the cytologic (Papanicolaou) smear may also prove negative.

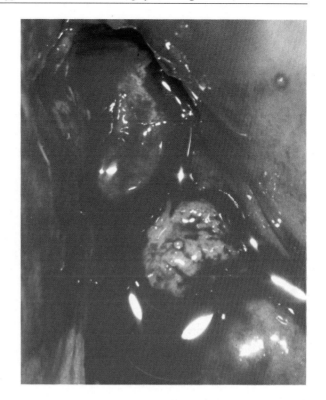

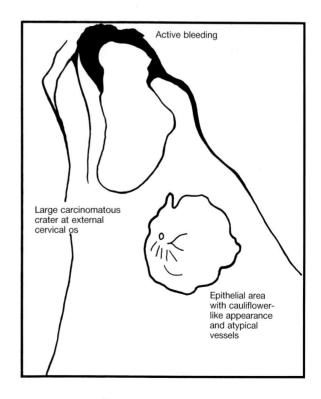

Active bleeding

Large carcinomatous crater at external cervical os

Epithelial area with cauliflower-like appearance and atypical vessels

Fig. 4.138: Carcinoma of cervical stump Ib

Patient: 63 years old, 16 years after subtotal hysterectomy. A large ulcer on the posterior cervical lip already suggests carcinoma on macroscopic inspection. The craterlike lesion shows vesicular structures and papillomatous areas with atypical vessels. In this case, too, the tissue is very fragile and bleeds easily. The Chrobak test was positive.

This patient had undergone a subtotal hysterectomy 16 years previously and had had no gynecologic examination since. At the time of examination she suffered from postmenopausal hemorrhage but had no other symptoms.

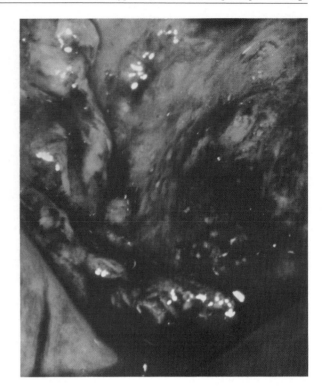

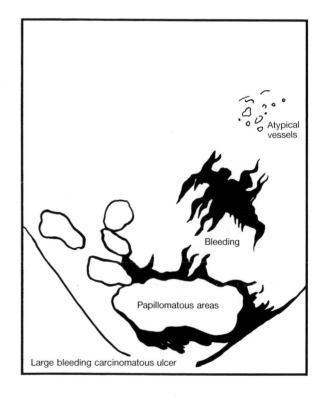

Fig. 4.139: Suspected carcinoma – hemorrhagic papillomatous endocervical tumor

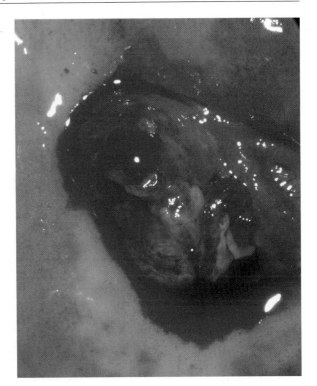

Patient: 50-year-old primipara. A large, very suspicious papillomatous hemorrhagic tumor is seen near the cervical canal. The surface appears partly necrotic and whitish, in the process of decaying.

Histologic findings: cervical carcinoma extending over the uterine cervix.

Cytologic finding: Papanicolaou smear IV.

The patient presented with irregular menopausal hemorrhaging but no other symptoms. A Wertheim-Meigs hysterectomy was performed with postoperative radiotherapy and high-dosage gestogen treatment. Followup observations have been made for 1.5 years.

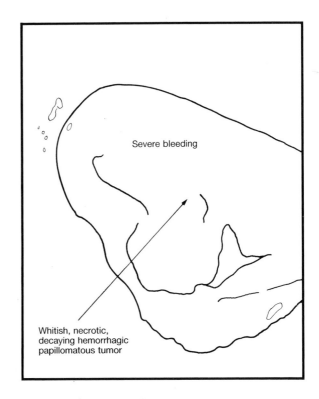

Severe bleeding

Whitish, necrotic, decaying hemorrhagic papillomatous tumor

Fig. 4.140: Vaginal carcinoma

Patient: 85 years old, pessary in place for 27 years. A round ulcer on the posterior vaginal wall has a large whitish area that is elevated and papillomatous. The tissue has a vesicular appearance and demonstrates numerous atypical vessels that tend to bleed easily. The Chrobak test is positive. The border of the carcinomatous ulcer has raised edges. Using a biopsy forceps, some of the friable tissue can be removed without difficulty for histologic confirmation.

This patient had been wearing a vaginal ring pessary for the past 27 years.

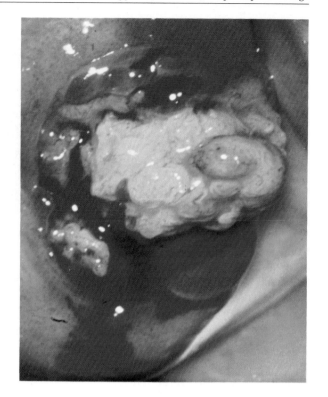

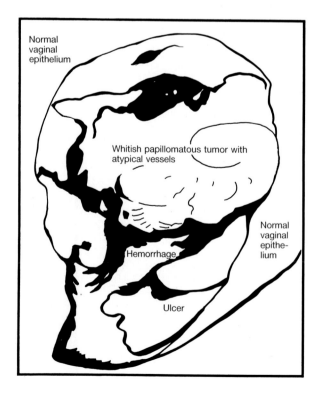

Fig. 4.141: Parametrial metastasis penetrating through vaginal wall after previous surgery for cervical carcinoma

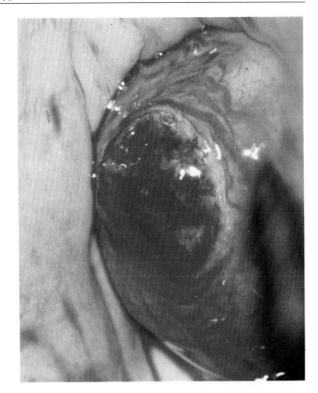

Patient: 41 years old, 5 years posthysterectomy.

A tumor, already macroscopically visible, appears in the left vaginal wall. The lesion has a large, round ulceration on the surface next to numerous atypical vessels. A marked bleeding tendency is noticeable owing to the fragile tissue, which also gave a positive Chrobak test.

A vaginal hysterectomy with right salpingo-oophorectomy had been performed 5 years previously. The histologic examination at that time revealed a microinvasive cervical carcinoma. When this metastasis was found the patient received intensive radiotherapy but died 3 years later.

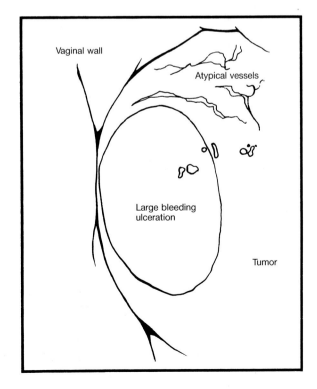

Fig. 4.142: Atypical vascularization following Wertheim-Meigs hysterectomy and postoperative radiotherapy for cervical carcinoma group I

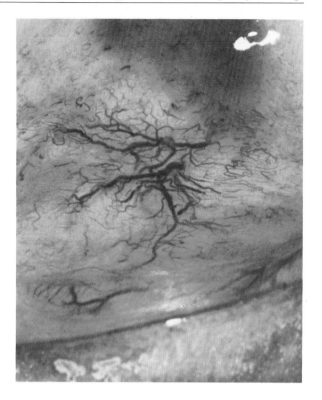

Numerous atypical vessels are present in the vaginal vault. The vascularization pattern can be regarded as hypertrophic, exhibiting a marked variety in caliber. There are also broken-off vessels with bizarre shapes and irregular courses.

This finding may cause difficulty in interpretation even for the experienced colposcopist. These vascular changes often develop after radiotherapy and do not necessarily indicate a malignant recurrence. Such cases are difficult to assess cytologically as well.

The patient, who had been treated by Wertheim-Meigs hysterectomy 6 years previously, has since died of metastases. Nevertheless, no local recurrence was detected.

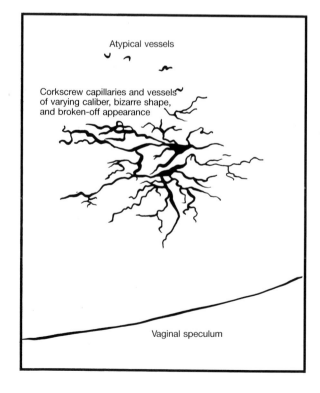

Atypical vessels

Corkscrew capillaries and vessels of varying caliber, bizarre shape, and broken-off appearance

Vaginal speculum

Fig. 4.143: Suspected carcinoma – exophytic changes

Patient: 50-year-old para 2. Whitish, polypoid, friable hemorrhagic tissue is seen welling out of the cervical canal. The Chrobak test is positive. The patient, in menopause, presented with complaint of irregular bleeding.
Cytologic finding: Papanicolaou V.
Histologic findings: highly differentiated uterine mucoid adenocarcinoma with a low mitosis rate and sparsely seen tumorous necrosis.

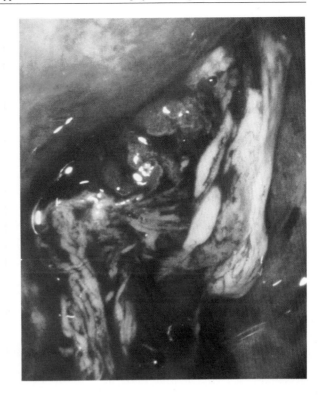

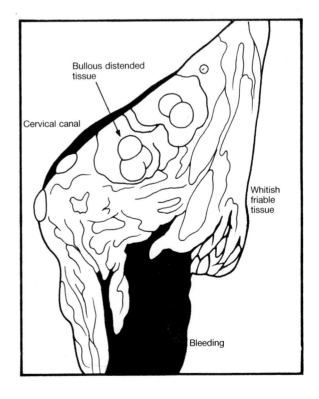

Fig. 4.144: Vaginal metastases of uterine carcinoma

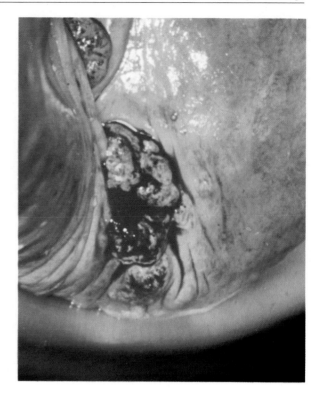

Patient: 53 years old, 2 years posthysterectomy. Several small papillomatous areas seen on the right side of the vaginal vault have atypical vessels and bleed on contact. The use of a metal sound indicates a positive Chrobak test. This lesion, which is rather small on macroscopic inspection, may easily be missed, particularly if a self-retaining speculum of the Cusco type is used. At first glance, such bleeding polypoid structures may be considered harmless granulation polyps. On colposcopic visualization, the tissue is seen to have an elevated and papillomatous appearance, and it turns white after application of acetic acid. Even more important, a small metastasis with marked atypical vessels becomes visible proximally.

The 53-year-old patient had undergone a total hysterectomy 2 years previously because of endometrial carcinoma.

Histologic clarification is always essential in such cases. Treatment consisted of local radiotherapy. Seven years later, there was a minor recurrence close to the introitus, near the posterior vaginal wall. This was simply removed by excision. (See Fig. 4.145.)

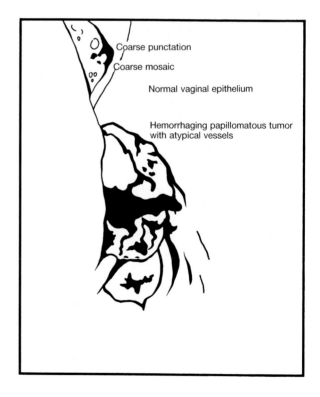

Coarse punctation

Coarse mosaic

Normal vaginal epithelium

Hemorrhaging papillomatous tumor with atypical vessels

**Fig. 4.145: Vaginal metasta-
ses near the posterior
vaginal wall**

Patient: same as in Fig. 4.144,
seven years later. Just posterior to the vaginal orifice near
the posterior vaginal wall one
can recognize two approximately pea-sized hemorrhagic
papillomatous tumors. The tissue is extremely friable, and
the surface of the larger tumor
presents a crater-like appearance.

Histologic findings: metastases of a middle grade differentiated adenocarcinoma in
the vaginal wall.

Followup colposcopic and cytologic examinations have
been performed at short intervals. No recurrence to date.

Pulmonary metastases ap-
peared sometime later.
Surgery was rejected because
both lungs were affected and
because the patient's cardiac
status was poor. The patient
has undergone numerous oxy-
gen treatments and chemo-
therapy (mistletoe) to date, but
the pulmonary situation appears unchanged. The subjective condition of the patient is
satisfactory overall. The
observation time totaled
18 years post-surgery,
16 years since the first recurrence, and 7 years since the
second relapse.

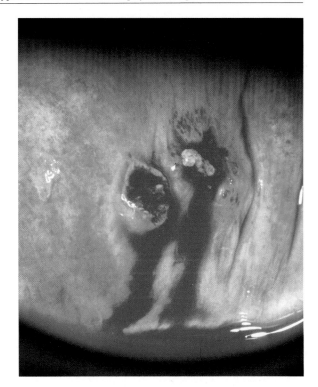

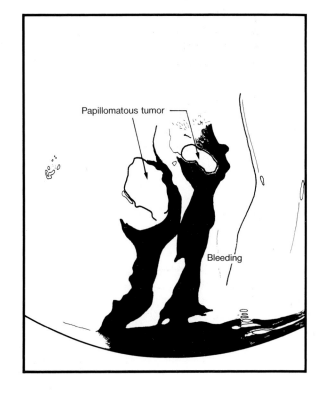

Papillomatous tumor

Bleeding

5: Comparison of Colposcopic, Cytologic, and Histologic Findings

To conclude this atlas I would like to demonstrate the limitations of colposcopy and cytology by means of three cases, including colposcopic, cytologic, and histologic color photodocumentation. Each method achieves excellent results, and it goes without saying that taking a cytologic smear for early detection of atypical epithelial changes requires much less experience than a colposcopic examination – one need only learn the technique of making a proper smear. Taking the cervical smear under colposcopic observation improves its quality and allows for a more accurate evelution; used together, these two methods optimize the chances that precursors and early stages of cervical carcinoma will be detected early. Apart from cancer detection, the importance of the clinical application of colposcopy lies in the evaluation of the numerous benign conditions at the cervix. This point cannot be overemphasized.

A histologic diagnosis was made in all cases with atypical findings. With the exception of the three presentations in this section, illustrations of histologic sections have been deliberately omitted so as not to interfere with the identification of colposcopic images. Besides, there are enough good textbooks available with plenty of histologic illustrations.

The experienced examiner working in private gyneocologic practice will not infrequently encounter diagnostic difficulties. These are inherent in both colposcopy and cytology. The ideal conditions of a large hospital where colposcopic, cytologic, and histologic examinations are carried out under one roof cannot always be applied to the routine of a daily practice. The cytologic smear may be taken by a younger physician who is inexperienced in performing a gynecologic examination. The smear is then sent to a large laboratory. The most common errors are described in Table 5.1.

I therefore consider it an advantage if the cytologic assessment can be done by the same person who performed the colposcopic examination and took the cervical smear. If both of these valuable examinations were conducted by the same examiner – which is rarely the case – one would achieve optimal diagnostic results. However, the obstacles to an accurate histologic evelution should not be underestimated. We all know that many pathology laboratories become overloaded when additional histologic sections from a conization specimen are requested.

Colposcopy has significant clinical value and should be incorporated into each

Table 5.1 Common Errors in Gynecologic Evaluation of the Cervix

Examiner errors
Inadequate smear specimen
Too little material
Taking sample from wrong site
Dried-up smear (owing to delayed fixation)
Incomplete colposcopic examination
Neglecting to apply 3% acetic acid solution
Failure even to perform a colposcopic examination
Cytologist errors
Poor staining
Inexperience or fatigue

gynecologic examination. Of course, accuracy in the detection of precursors and early stages of cervical carcinoma becomes limited when atypical epithelium cannot be visualized because of its presence in the endocervical canal (as demonstrated in Case 3). In a case like this, colposcopy and cytology are especially complementary.

As many instances in this atlas illustrate, even the experienced colposcopist may encounter diagnostic difficulties. This is especially the case with the atypical transformation zone and with inflammatory conditions. In such cases it is advisable to make frequent use of directed punch biopsies, which should be taken under colposcopic visualization employing a special biopsy forceps. The excised specimen should be large enough to supply the pathologist with adequate material for a definitive diagnosis. This technique of colposcopically directed punch biopsy is now widely practiced.

In the following examples, *Case I* shows agreement of the colposcopic picture with the cytologic and histologic findings. In *Case 2,* the cytologic smear did not correspond with the histologic picture, whereas the colposcopic and histologic findings were in agreement. In *Case 3,* the colposcopic findings were not confirmed by histology, whereas the cytologic and histologic pictures corresponded.

Comment: Case 1 (Figs. 5.1 through 5.5)

Colposcopic findings (Figs. 5.1 through 5.3): Coarse mosaic and coarse punctation (suspicion of carcinoma in situ)
Cytologic findings (Fig. 5.4):
Papanicolaou test positive IVa (suspected carcinoma in situ)
Histologic findings: Carcinoma in situ – CIN III

This example represents the ideal concept: The colposcopically observed coarse mosaic and punctation give a clear indication of histologic atypia. The cytologic examination already suggested carcinoma in situ – CIN III. I would like to emphasize, however, that premalignant epithelial changes cannot always be demonstrated from the colposcopic image as unequivocally as in this case. Time and again the examiner will be confronted with situations in which atypical colposcopic findings are difficult to assess, as for example in the presence of inflammation or in cases of atrophy.

It is important that the colposcopic findings be classified as suspicious and that negative cytologic findings also be histologically clarified. This is best accomplished by taking directed biopsies under colposcopic observation – a point repeatedly stressed in this text. The procedure causes little discomfort for the patient and can be performed on an outpatient basis. The criteria for colposcopic findings that require biopsy are listed in Table 1.2.

Case 1: Agreement of Colposcopic, Cytologic, and Histologic Findings
(Fig. 5.1 through 5.5)

These findings were diagnosed in a 42-year-old woman para 4 (no complications) during a routine examination for early detection of cancer. The Pap test was IVa (carcinoma in situ). A total vaginal uterine prolapse made it necessary to perform a vaginal hysterectomy with anterior and posterior plasty.

Colposcopic Findings
(Figs. 5.1 and 5.2)

Fig. 5.1: Before application of 3% acetic acid. Coarse mosaic and coarse punctation are seen near the anterior cervical os; the findings are less evident at the posterior cervical os. The very obvious colposcopic changes, recognizable even without the application of 3% acetic acid, indicate a severe dysplasia or carcinoma in situ.

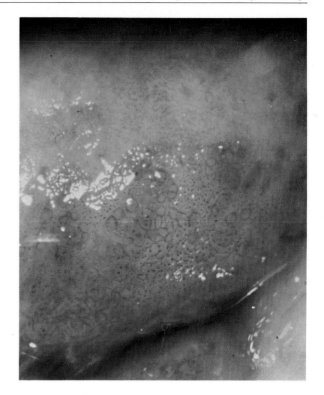

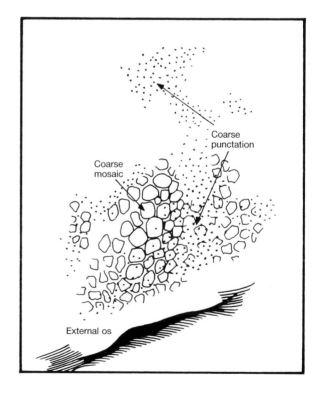

Fig. 5.2: After application of 3% acetic acid. Coarse mosaic and coarse punctation in white epithelium. The atypical findings are even more easily recognizable. In addition, several gland openings with white keratotic rims are now visible.

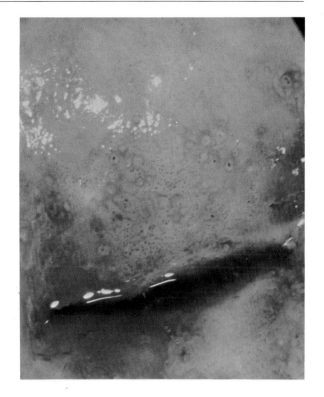

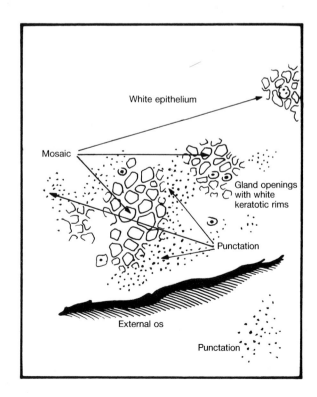

Cytologic Findings (Fig. 5.3)

Figure 5.3: Papanicolaou smear IVa suspicious of carcinoma in situ – CIN III.

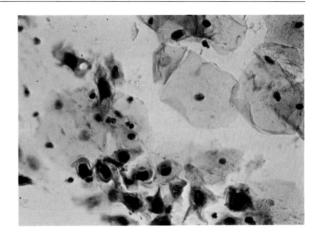

Histologic Findings (Figs. 5.4 and 5.5)

Fig. 5.4: Carcinoma in situ – CIN III (approximately ×80 magnification).

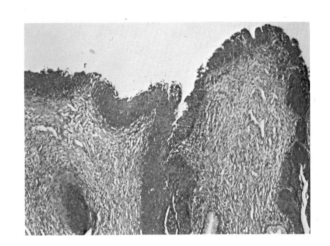

Fig. 5.5: Carcinoma in situ – CIN III (approximately ×80 magnification).

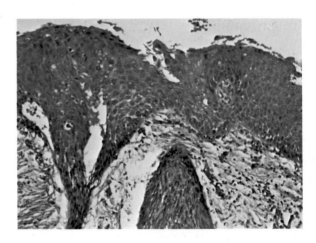

Comment (Figs. 5.6 through 5.8)

Colposcopic findings (Fig. 5.6): papillomatous area with coarse punctation and erosion (suspicious of carcinoma in situ)

Cytologic findings (Fig. 5.7): Papanicolaou smear negative, II

Histologic findings (Fig. 5.8): Carcinoma in situ – CIN III

In this case, the initially examining physician, who took the cytologic smear, performed no colposcopic examination. The result of the cytologic evaluation done by a remote laboratory was Papanicolaou II (negative).

Four weeks later the patient was incidentally seen at my office where changes suspicious of carcinoma in situ could be identified with the colposcope, as shown in Fig. 5.6.

It is difficult to incorporate these findings into the classification scheme, and I have placed the lesion under the heading papillomatous tumor (suspicious of carcinoma). Fortunately, the histologic findings confirmed carcinoma in situ – CIN III.

The reader will realize how complicated judgement may become and that the final decision depends on the personal approach of the examiner. As regards the management of such a case, I do not consider the classification to be important; it *is* essential for the colposcopist to regard this as a conditionally premalignant or malignant condition and to initiate histologic clarification.

In this case a colposcopically directed punch biopsy indicated the presence of carcinoma in situ, and the hysterectomy specimen confirmed the diagnosis once more on histologic examination.

This example is by no means exceptional. It merely demonstrates the vital importance of combining colposcopy and cytology as complementary methods in the diagnosis of early malignancy.

Case 2: Difference Between Colposcopic and Cytologic Findings (Failure of Cytology) (Figs. 5.6 through 5.8)

The patient, a 50-year-old primipara, had a 4-year history of oral contraceptive use. She presented with no symptoms.

Colposcopic Findings (Fig. 5.6)

Papilloma with coarse punctation and erosion (suspicious of carcinoma in situ). A large papillomatous lesion is seen on the anterior cervical lip, exhibiting coarse punctation, areas of erosion, and a bleeding tendency. The border of the cervical canal cannot be visualized.

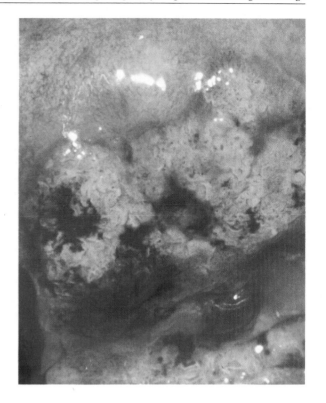

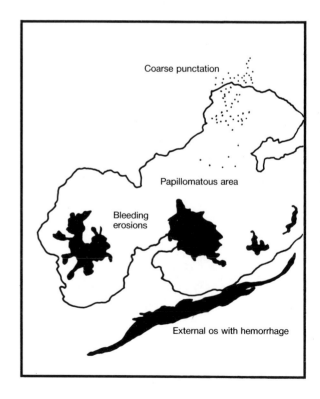

Coarse punctation

Papillomatous area

Bleeding erosions

External os with hemorrhage

Cytologic Findings (Fig. 5.7)

Papanicolaou test negative, II.

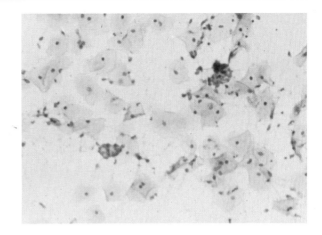

Histologic Findings (Fig. 5.8)

Carcinoma in situ – CIN III (approximately 80× magnification).

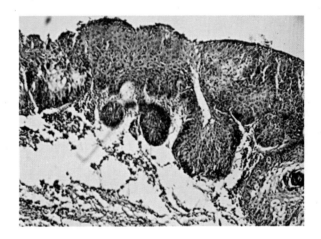

Comment (Figs. 5.9 through 5.11)

Colposcopic findings (Fig. 5.9): Original squamous epithelium

Cytologic findings (Fig. 5.10): Papanicolaou test positive, IV (suspicion of carcinoma in situ)

Histologic findings (Fig. 5.11): Endocervical carcinoma in situ — CIN III

I have pointed out several times that the value of the colposcopic examination is limited when atypical epithelial changes are not observable, that is, when they lie in the endocervical canal. This is the situation in Case 3. On the basis of the positive Papanicolaou test, a conization was performed. The histologic evaluation indicates a carcinoma in situ — CIN III (Fig. 5.11). Treatment was continued in another clinic. Conization was repeated and the histologic diagnosis endocervical carcinoma in situ was confirmed. Since the patient suffered from chronic pelvic inflammatory disease with adnexal masses, a hysterectomy with bilateral salpingo-oophorectomy was performed.

Like Case 2, this example demonstrates the importance of colposcopy and cytology as complementary methods. The colposcopic finding, original squamous epithelium, is in this case insufficient for a diagnosis, since the squamocolumnar epithelial junction was not observable. Such findings have to be recorded as "no evaluation possible."

We do know that the occurrence of atypical epithelium within the endocervical canal is rare in women of childbearing age. GLATTHAAR reports an incidence of 2.8%. Other authors give a higher incidence ranging from 5 to 15%. For routine examination in daily practice, however, it is of minor importance what percentage of atypical epithelium will be found endocervically. *The critical point is that such a condition exists, and colposcopy and cytology should therefore be applied in conjunction with each other.*

Case 3: Colposcopic and Cytologic Findings Differ (Colposcopy Inconclusive) (Figs. 5.9 through 5.11)

This patient, a 39-year-old nullipara, presented for routine examination. She had no symptoms.

Colposcopic Findings (Fig. 5.9)

Squamous epithelium – squamocolumnar epithelial juncture not observable. Since the squamocolumnar epithelial junction could not be visualized, the findings were recorded as "no evaluation possible." Minimal contact bleeding occurred after the cervical smear was taken.

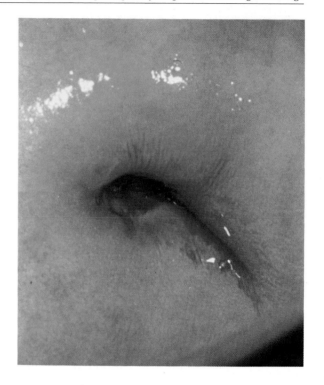

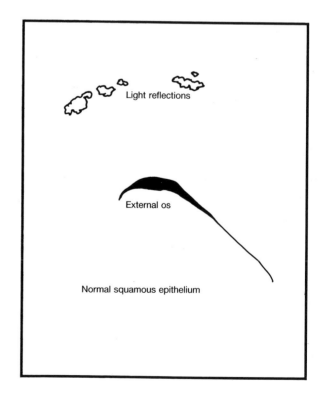

Cytologic Finding (Fig. 5.10)

Papanicolaou smear IV, suspicion of carcinoma in situ – CIN III.

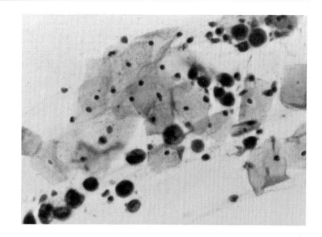

Histologic Findings (Fig. 5.11)

Endocervical carcinoma in situ – CIN III (approximately ×80 magnification).

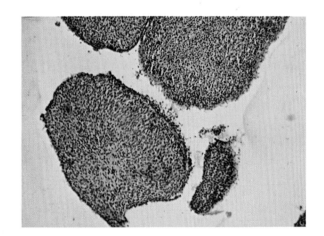

6: References

Monographs and Books

BERGMANN U. Kolposkopische Bilder in heutiger Sicht. Ein Atlas für die gynäkologische Praxis. Berlin: Akademie-Verlag; 1979.

BOLTEN K. Introduction to Colposcopy. New York: Grune and Stratton; 1960.

BURKE L. Colposcopy in Clinical Practice. Philadelphia: F. A. Davis; 1977.

CARTIER R. Atlas d'Endoscopie, Colposcopie. Paris: Laboratoires Roussel; 1975.

CARTIER R. Colposcopie Pratique. Basel: Karger; 1977.

COPPLESON M., E. PIXLEY, B. REID. Colposcopy, a Scientific and Practical Approach to the Cervix in Health and Disease. Springfield IL.: C. C. Thomas; 1971.

COUPEZ F., J. M. CARRERA, S. DEXEUS. Traité et Atlas de Colposcopie. Paris: Masson; 1974.

CRAMER H., G. OHLY. Die Kolposkopie in der Praxis. 3rd ed. Stuttgart: Thieme; 1975.

GANSE R. Kolpofotogramme. Berlin: Akademie-Verlag; 1953 (vols 1 and 2), 1955 (vol 3).

GANSE R. Das normale und pathologische Gefäßbild der Portio vaginalis uteri. Berlin: Akademie-Verlag; 1958.

GLATTHAAR E. Kolposkopie. In: SEITZ L., AMREICH I., eds. Biologie und Pathologie des Weibes. Vol 3, p 911. Munich: Urban & Schwarzenberg; 1955.

GRIMMER H. Gut- und bösartige Erkrankungen der Vulva. Vol 1. Berlin: Grosse Verlag; 1974.

HIERSCHE H.-D. Funktionelle Morphologie des fetalen und kindlichen cervicalen Drüsenfeldes im Uterus. Ergebnisse der Anatomie und Entwicklungsgeschichte. Berlin: Springer; 1970.

HINSELMANN H. Aktuelle Probleme der praktischen und wissenschaftlichen Kolposkopie. Jena: VEB Gustav Fischer; 1956.

HINSELMANN H. Die Ätiologie, Symptomatologie und Diagnostik des Uteruskarzinoms. In: VEIT I., W. STOCKEL, eds. Handbuch der Gynäkologie. 3rd ed. Vol 6, p 845. Munich: Bergmann; 1930.

JORDAN J. A., A. SINGER. The Cervix. Philadelphia: W. B. Saunders; 1976.

KERN G. Carcinoma in situ. Berlin: Springer; 1964.

KERN G. Diagnostik des Zervixkarzinoms. Gynäk Geburtsh 3: 449; 1972.

KERN G., E. KERN-BONTKE. Ektropium der Zervixschleimhaut (Pseudoerosion, Umwandlungszone, Erythroplakie). Gynäk Geburtsh 3: 153; 1972.

KINDERMANN G., K. G. OBER. Ausbreitung des Zervixkarzinoms. Gynäk Geburtsh 3: 432; 1972.

KOLSTAD P., A. STAFL. Atlas of Colposcopy. Oslo-Bergen-Tromcs: Universitetsforlaget; 1972.

KOLSTAD P., A. STAFL: Atlas der Kolposkopie. Stuttgart: Enke; 1983.

KORTING G. W. Praktische Dermatologie der Genitalregion. Stuttgart: Schattauer; 1980.

LANGLEY F. A., A. C. CROMPTON. Epithelial Abnormalities of the Cervix Uteri. New York: Springer; 1973.

LIMBURG H. Tumoren der Vagina. Gynäk Geburtsh 3: 321; 1972.

LIMBURG H. Tumoren der Vulva. Gynäk Geburtsh 3: 335; 1972.

MADEJ J. Kolposkopia. Warsaw: Pans stwoy Zaklad Wydawnictw Lekarskich; 1982.

MESTWERDT G., R. MOLL, D. WAGNER-KOLB, H. J. WESPI. Atlas der Kolposkopie. 5th ed. Stuttgart: G. Fisher; 1980.

PERONI M. Colposcopia E Fisiopatologia Cervico-Vaginale. Edito a curadella. Poli industria chimica – divisione Medica 1983.

RIBBERT H., H. HAMPERL. Lehrbuch der allgemeinen Pathologie und der pathologischen Anatomie. Berlin: Vogel; 1940.

RIEPER J. P., C. SALGADO, L. R. SANCHES. Colposcopia. Fename – Fundacão nacional de material escolar. Ministero de Educacão e Cultura; 1970.

RIEPER J. P. Patologia Cervical. Colposcopia, Citologia, Histologia. São Paulo: Manole; 1978.

SCOTT J. W. Stereocolposcopic Atlas of the Uterine Cervix. Kendall, FL: Zephyr; 1971.

SEIDL ST. Kolposkopie. Befunde der Portio, der Vagina und der Vulva. Eine Dia-Sammlung mit Begleittext. Basel: Rocom F. Hoffmann-La Roche; 1979.

SEIDL ST. Praktische Karzinom-Frühdiagnostik in der Gynäkologie. Stuttgart: Thieme; 1974.

SCHAETZING A. E. The Colposcopical Parameters of Dysplasia and Carcinoma in Situ of the Uterine Cervix. Monograph presented for the degree of Doctor of Philosophy in Medicine at the University of Stellenbosch, Republic of South Africa; 1981.

THOMSEN K., W. HUMKE. Entzündungen der Vagina. Gynäk Geburtsh. 3: 54; 1972.

THOMSEN K., W. HUMKE. Entzündungen der Vulva. Gynäk Geburtsh 3: 66. Stuttgart: Thieme; 1972.

WESPI H. J. Entstehung und Früherfassung des Portiokarzinoms. Basel: Schwabe; 1946.

Selected Papers and Articles

AHERN J. K. Colposcopy and Private Practice. Gyne-med. INC Palo Alto, CA: GyneMed, Inc; 1973.

ALMENDRAL A. C., G. SZALMAY, L. JOCHUM, H. MÜL-LER. Vor- und Frühstadien des Zervixkarzinoms. Fortschr Med 92: 1007; 1974.

ANDRÝS J., K. VÁCHA, M. ROSOL, J. KOPEĆNY: Präkanzerosen der Cervix uteri in der Schwangerschaft. Zbl Gynäk 96: 1012; 1974.

ARNS H. H. Krebsverdächtige Veränderungen der Portio uteri und ihre kolpophotographische Darstellung unter besonderer Berücksichtigung der Gefäße. Krebsarzt 17: 197; 1962.

ARNS H. H. Das Karzinom der Portio uteri in der gynäkologischen Praxis. Krebsarzt 16: 156; 1961.

BAADER O. 12 Jahre Karzinom-Diagnostik in gynäkologischer Praxis. Geburtsh Frauenheilk 24: 402; 1964.

BAADER O. Zur Diagnostik des Genitalkarzinoms in der gynäkologischen Praxis. Fortschr Med 88: 476; 1970.

BAADER O. Frühdiagnostik und Prävention des Zervixkarzinoms in der Praxis. Dtsch Ärztebl 66: 411; 1969.

BAADER O. Pilleneffekte an der Portio vaginalis uteri. Dtsch Ärztebl 73: 2851; 1976.

BAADER O. Kolposkopische Bilder bei Jugendlichen. Presented at the 4th conference of the Association for Study of the Uterine Cervix, April 12 – 15, 1978. Cited in Geburtsh Frauenheilk 38: 678; 1978.

BAADER O. Kolposkopie des Kondyloms und Papilloms. Presented at the 5th Conference of the Society for the Study of the Uterine Cervix, April 19 – 23, 1980. Cited in Geburtsh Frauenheilk 41: 71; 1981.

BACHMANN F. F. Das Rezidiv des Ca in situ der Zervix. Geburtsh Frauenheilk 32: 678; 1972.

BACHMANN F., K. HEINERICH. Zur Klinik und Therapie des beginnenden Karzinoms der Zervix. Med Welt 23: 1536; 1972.

BAJARDI F. Histologische Diagnose von Vor- und Frühstadien des Gebärmutterhalskrebses. Ost Z Erforsch Bekämpf Krebskrh 27: 101; 1970.

BAJARDI F. Spontanregression des pathologischen Gebärmutterhalsepithels im histologischen Bild. Ost Z Erforsch Bekämpf Krebskrh 27: 1; 1972.

BAJARDI F. Zur Frage des kombinierten Einsatzes von Kolposkopie und Zytologie. Frauenarzt 20: 186; 1979.

BAJARDI F. Das Verhalten von Epithel und Stroma beim frühinvasiven Zervixkarzinom. Presented at the 5th conference of the Society for the Study of the Uterine Cervix, April 19–23, 1980. Cited in Geburtsh Frauenheilk 41: 68; 1981.

BAJARDI F. Histologische Abklärung der pathologischen Zervixzytologie – Ergebnis der Kleinbiopsie und der Konisation. Ninth Seminar in Clinical Cytology, Munich, December 6–12, 1987.

BAJARDI F., H. KASTNER. Über den Aussagewert des pathologischen Zellbefundes im Rahmen großer gynäkologischer Programme. Wien klin Wschr 84: 633; 1972.

BAUER HK. Die Sanierung der Portio uteri mit Albothyl als Krebsprophylaxe in der ambulanten Praxis (Dokumentation der Befunde mit Farb-Kolpofotografie). Medizinische 10: 1645; 1959.

BAUER HK. Über den gegenwärtigen Stand der Diagnostik und Therapie des weiblichen Genitalkarzinoms. Hess Ärztebl 29: 552; 1968.

BAUER HK. Langzeitbeobachtungen bei atypischem Epithel (nach einem Vortrag auf dem 5. Weltkongress für Gynäkologie und Geburtshilfe in Sydney 1967). Med Welt 19(NF): 2048; 1968.

BAUER HK. Die Bedeutung der Kolposkopie bei der Frühdiagnostik des Kollumkarzinoms in der täglichen Praxis. Frauenarzt 11: 200; 1970.

BAUER HK. Zur Problematik falsch negativer zytologischer Befunde. Geburtsh Frauenheilk 31: 572; 1971.

BAUER HK. Kolposkopie. Diagnostik 5: 528; 1972.

BAUER HK. Die Bedeutung der kolpofotografischen Dokumentation bei Langzeitbeobachtungen von dysplastischem Epithel der Cervix uteri. Presentation at the First Workshop of the Association for the Study of the Uterine Cervix, 1972. Mitteilungsdienst der Gesellschaft zur Bekämpfung der Krebskrankheiten Nordrhein-Westfalen. 6: 939; 1973.

BAUER HK. Dysplasia and Ca in situ of young patients; colposcopic and cytological observations of the courses. Presented at the Sixth Clinical Meeting of the American Society for Colposcopy and Colpomicroscopy, 1973. J Reprod Med (Chicago) 5; 1974.

BAUER HK. Die Kolposkopie als Werkzeug gynäkologischer Diagnostik. Selecta 9: 804; 1974.

BAUER HK. Colposcopy. Documentation of Colposcopic Findings – Their Clinical and Practical Significance. Presented at the Second Curso Congreso de Patologia cervical, May 1, 1975, in Valencia, Spain.

BAUER HK. Kolposkopische Kriterien der atypischen Umwandlungszone. Presented at the Third Conference of the Association for the Study of the Uterine Cervix, May 1–5, 1970, in Wiesbaden.

BAUER HK. Kolposkopie. Arch Gynäk 214: 240; 1973.

BAUER HK. Zur Frage einer Vereinfachung der Nomenklatur bei der Kolposkopie. Frauenarzt 13: 137; 1972.

BAUER HK. Remarks concerning VON RUMMEL H. H., R. FRICK, D. HEBERLING, D. SCHUBERT. Verlaufskontrolle bei Patientinnen mit suspekter Zytologie (Papanicolaou III D). Geburtsh Frauenheilk 37: 521; 1977, Geburtsh Frauenheilk 38: 396, 1978.

BAUER HK. Kolposkopie: Gerätevergleich, Hilfsmethoden und Befunde. Diagnostik 10: 13; 1977.

BAUER HK. Kolposkopie im Zeitalter der Zytologie noch zeitgemäß? Frauenarzt 19: 134; 1978.

BAUER HK. Die Kolposkopie und ihre Bedeutung als eine frühdiagnostische Methode für die gynäkologische Untersuchung. Med Welt 29: 1713; 1978.

BAUER HK. Observations of the course of colposcopic atypical epithelium (observations over 20 years). Presented at the Third World Congress for Cervical Pathology and Colposcopy, Orlando, FL, 1978.

BAUER HK. Über die Aussagekraft von kolposkopischem und zytologischem Befund bei der Früherkennungsuntersuchung der Frau – Ergebnisse einer Gemeinschaftsstudie über 923 Fälle. Presented at the Fifth Conference of the Association for the Study of the Uterine Cervix, Wiesbaden, 1980. Med Welt 32: 414; 1981.

BAUER HK. Die Bedeutung der Kolposkopie und ihre Aufgaben in Klinik und Praxis. Speculum (Geburtshilfe – Frauenheilkunde – Strahlenheilkunde – Forschung – Konsequenzen) Wien 1: 3–8; 1983.

BAUER HK. Development and regression of atypical cervical epithelium as documented by sequential colour colpophotographs, the cervix and the lower female genital tract. Milano, Italy, 3: 275–282; 1985.

BAUER HK. Kolposkopie bei der Abklärung dysplastischer Zervixveränderungen unverzichtbar. Gynecol 8: 49–52; 1987.

BAUER HK. Funktionskolposkopie – diagnostische Möglichkeiten der Kolposkopie. Frauenarzt 29: 161–165; 1988.

BAUER HK. The importance of colposcopy in detection of viral infections at the cervix. In: The Cervix and the Lower Female Tract. Vol 6. Milan: 1988. In press.

BAYRLE W. Kritische Betrachtungen zur Rate der "falschnegativen" Befunde in der gynäkologischen Zytologie. Geburtsh Frauenheilk 37: 864; 1977.

BERGER J. Die Entwicklung der neuzeitlichen Karzinom-Diagnostik in der Gynäkologie seit der Jahrhundertwende. Gynäkologia 166: 85; 1968.

BERGLEITHER R., H. BETTZIECHE. Klinische und kolposkopische Befunde bei Präkanzerosen der Zervix uteri – ein Beitrag zur Wertigkeit einer Auswahlzytologie. Zbl Gynäk 97: 12; 1975.

BERIĆ B., H. SMOLKA. Über den Einfluß der in der Kolposkopie angewandten Reagenzien auf das Zellbild des Portioabstriches. Geburtsh Frauenheilk 18: 852; 1958.

BETTENDORF U. Strahlenbedingte Veränderungen des Vaginal- and Portioepithels. Zbl Gynäk 11: 689–697; 1979.

BETTENDORF U., D. HEERKLOTZ. Virusinfektionen der Cervix uteri: Herpes simplex genitalis und Condylomata acuminata. Deutsch Ärzteblatt 80: 27–29; 1983.

BISCH E., M. MÜLLER. Studien an Praecancerosen der Mundschleimhaut und Vulva mit Hilfe des Kolposkops. Roche Medizinischer Bilddienst, 1960.

BOLTEN K. Practical colposcopy in early cervical and vaginal cancer. 5: 808; 1968.

BOSCHANN H.-W. Kolposkopie. Z ärztl Fortbild 52: 3; 1963.

BOWIEN H. Erfahrungen und Ergebnisse unserer Krebsberatungsstelle während der Jahre 1948 bis 1952 mit Vorschlägen zur Beseitigung organisatorischer Mängel in der Krebsprophylaxe. Geburtsh Frauenheilk 13: 796; 1953.

BRANDL K., V. GRÜNBERGER. Der Wert verschiedener Spezialuntersuchungen für die Beurteilung makroskopisch unverdächtiger Erosionen. Geburtsh Frauenheilk 14: 434; 1954.

BRANDL K., V. GRÜNBERGER. Weitere Resultate ambulanter Erosionsuntersuchungen. Geburtsh Frauenheilk 17: 352; 1957.

BRANDL K., E. KOFLER. Die Krebsfrüherkennungsmethoden bei 230 Fällen mit Kollumkarzinom. Geburtsh Frauenheilk 19: 415; 1959.

BREDLAND R. Kolposkopische Diagnose der gynäkologischen Trichomoniasis. Geburtsh Frauenheilk 25: 815; 1965.

BREINL H. Fraglicher Wert der Kolposkopie als Methode zur Fahndung nach dem Kollumkarzinom. Dtsch Ärztebl 67: 1455; 1970.

BREINL H., F. DENHARD, J. WILHELM. Intensivierte Frühdiagnostik des Gebärmutterhalskarzinoms. Minerva ginec (Torino) 23: 86; 1971.

BRETT A. J., F. COUPEZ. Colposcopie. Encyclopedie Medico-Chirugicale. (Paris) 60: 1–11; 1969.

BRUNTSCH K. H. Zur Problematik der feingeweblichen Diagnostik früher Plattenepithelkarzinomstadien des Gebärmutterhalses (mit einem Vorschlag zur Erkundung der prospektiven Bedeutung "verdächtiger Epithelbildungen"). Geburtsh Frauenheilk 18: 238; 1948.

BUCKWAR U. Zur Organisation kolposkopischer Vorsichtsuntersuchungen. Dtsch Gesundh Wes 15: 312; 1960.

BÜTTNER H. H. Histologie der Vorstadien des Zervixkarzinoms. Z ärztl Fortbild 66: 1244; 1972.

BÜTTNER H. H., H. KYANK, G. BADER. Histologische Nomenklatur und Einteilung der gutartigen Epithelveränderungen an der Cervix uteri und der Vor- und Frühstadien des Zervixkarzinoms. Zbl Gynäk 96: 961; 1974.

BUSCH W. Die Stellung der Kolposkopie im Rahmen der Frühdiagnostik praemaligner und maligner Zervixepithelveränderungen. Presented at the Eighth Conference of the Association for the Study of the Uterine Cervix, 1986.

COPPLESON M. Die Stellung der Kolposkopie bei der Entdeckung und Behandlung des Ca in situ der Zervix. J Obstet Gynecol Brit Cwlth 71: 854; 1964.

COPPLESON M., L. REID, A. SINGER. The process of cervical regeneration after electrocauterization. Part 1. Histological and colposcopic study. Part 2. Histochemical, autoradiographic, and pH study. Aust N Z J Obstet Gynaecol 7: 125; 1967.

COUPEZ F. La place de la colposcopie dans l'examen gynecologique actuel. Rev franc Gynec 65: 209; 1970.

CRAMER H. Aussprache zu "kolpofotografische Demonstration" von A. SCHMITT. Geburtsh Frauenheilk 14: 86; 1954.

CRAMER H. Die neuen Wege der gynäkologischen Krebsfrühdiagnostik und ihre Erfolgsaussichten. Medizinische 5: 642; 1954.

CRAMER H. Ein weiterer technischer Fortschritt in der Kolpofotografie. Cited in Geburtsh Frauenheilk 15: 665; 1955.

CRAMER H. Kritisches zum Begriff der sogenannten atypischen Umwandlungszone. Geburtsh Frauenheilk 21: 706; 1961.

CRAMER H. Symposium über angewandte exfoliative Zytologie. Cited in Geburtsh Frauenheilk 18: 97; 1958.

CRAMER H., E. LIND. Die endozervikale Lokalisation des Karzinoms und sog. Oberflächenkarzinoms am Gebärmutterhals unter diagnostischen Gesichtspunkten. Geburtsh Frauenheilk 22: 161; 1962.

CRAMER H., G. SCHULTE. Kolposkopische Photographie im Agfa-Color-Negativ-Positiv-Verfahren. Geburtsh Frauenheilk 13: 212; 1953.

DIETEL H., A. FOCKEN. Das Schicksal des atypischen Epithels an der Portio. Geburtsh Frauenheilk 15: 593; 1955.

DOHNAL V. Schwangerschaft und Schleimhautveränderungen an der Cervix uteri. Geburtsh Frauenheilk 27: 392; 1967.

DOHNAL V. Neue Aspekte in der Kolposkopie und Zytologie. M. D. G. B. K. 36: 17–23; 1980.

DOHNAL V., L. KOTAL. Über die idealplattenepithelbedeckte Portio vaginalis uteri und ihre Beziehung zu Fortpflanzungsfunktionen. Geburtsh Frauenheilk 27: 485–492; 1967.

EISEN K. Kolposkopie in der täglichen Praxis. Cited in Geburtsh Frauenheilk 15: 762; 1955.

FOCKEN A. Rationelle Anwendung von Kolposkopie und Cytologie in der Frühdiagnostik des Kollum-Karzinoms. Med Welt 15: 2070; 1955.

FOCKEN A., G. FRANZ. Carcinoma in situ und Schwangerschaft. Geburtsh Frauenheilk 16: 790; 1956.

FRANKEN H. Das Kolpolux, ein einfaches Gerät zum Kolposkopieren in der allgemeinen Sprechstunde. Geburtsh Frauenheilk 17: 803; 1957.

FRANKEN H. Präventivmaßnahmen zur Bekämpfung des Gebärmutterkrebses. Münch Med Wschr 99: 1014; 1957.

FRITSCH K. Befunde bei gezielten Probeexzisionen an der Portio. Med Mschr 12: 817; 1960.

FRITSCH K. Über Endozervixkolposkopie. Geburtsh Frauenheilk 19: 64; 1959.

FROMMOLT G. Zur Dokumentation von Portiobefunden. Zbl Gynäk 83: 347; 1961.

GANSE R. Die Prophylaxe des Portiokarzinoms. Z proph Med 8: 187; 1956.

GANSE R. Zur Klinik des Microcarcinoms. GBK Mitteilungsdienst 5: 565; 1969.

GANSE R. Gefäßneubildung beim präinvasiven und fertigen Karzinom. Geburtsh Frauenheilk 20: 694; 1960.

GANSE R. Veränderungen der atypischen Gefäße des Portiokarzinoms unter Telecobaltbestrahlung. Geburtsh Frauenheilk 27: 476; 1967.

GANSE R., R. KRIMMENAU, J. BREY. Papillomatose Veränderungen der Portio und deren carcinomatöse Potenz. Geburtsh Frauenheilk 22: 232; 1962.

GISSMANN L. Human papillomaviruses as an essential factor for the development of cervical cancer. (Pers. Mitteilung). In press.

GÖRCS J., I. BREILA, F. HARGITAI. Über die Progression der Praeblastomatosen colli uteri. Minerva Ginec 23: 82; 1971.

GRIMMER H. Morbus Bowen. Z Haut Geschl Kr 44: 21–28; 1969.

GRIMMER H. Multizentrischer Morbus Bowen der Vulva. Z Haut Geschl Kr 43: 173–177; 1968.

GRÜNBERGER V. Prophylaxe des Collumcarcinoms durch Elektrokoagulation der Erythroplakie. Minerva Ginec 23: 178; 1971.

GRÜNBERGER V. Prophylaxe und Frühdiagnose des Kollumkarzinoms. Wien Klin Wschr 90 (19): 677; 1978.

GUHR O. Hormonal induzierte Portioveränderungen unter Ovulationshemmern. Münch Med Wschr 114: 766; 1972.

GUHR O. Portioveränderungen unter Kortikosteroiden. Münch Med Wschr 115: 1020; 1973.

GUHR O. Kolposkopische, zytologische und histologische Portiobefunde bei ovulationshemmenden Medikamenten. Arch Gynäk 202: 205; 1965.

HÄRTER G. Gynäkologische Vorsorgeuntersuchungen in einer Landpraxis. Fortschr Med 92: 1297; 1974.

HAMPERL H. Gestalt und Struktur der Portio vaginalis uteri zu verschiedenen Lebensaltern. Geburtsh Frauenheilk 25: 289–298; 1965.

HAMPERL H., C. KAUFMANN, K. G. OBER. Das Problem der Malignität unter besonderer Berücksichtigung des Carcinoma in situ an der Cervix uteri. Klin Wschr 32: 825; 1954.

HARTMANN G., H. LAU. Zur Diagnostik bei Vorstadien und Frühformen des Zervixkarzinoms am kommunalen Klinikum. Zbl Gynäk 95: 614; 1973.

HASEGAWA T., ET AL. Quantitive analysis of the whiteness of the atypical cervical transformation zone. J Reprod Med 30: 773–776; 1985.

HASELHORST G. Zur Frage des Wesens der Portioleukoplakien. Geburtsh Gynäk 98: 526; 1930.

HASELHORST G. Portioleukoplakie und Karzinom. Geburtsh Gynäk 101: 622; 1932.

HEINZL F. Überwachung von Dysplasien. Gynäkologie 14: 212–216; 1981.

HEINZL F. Die kolposkopische Beurteilung der Zervix uteri nach Behandlung einer CIN Grad III mittels Konisation, Kryochirurgie oder CO_2 Laser-Therapie. Presented at the Sixth Conference of the Association for the Study of the Uterine Cervix, Wiesbaden, 1982.

HELD E. Der heutige Stand der Prophylaxe und der Frühdiagnose des Kollumkarzinoms. Cited at the First Conference of the Association for the Study of the Uterine Cervix, Wiesbaden, 1972. GBK Mitteilungsdienst 6: 807; 1973.

HERBECK G. Das Carcinoma in situ der Portio bei der Frau unter 30 Jahren. Med Welt 27 (N F): 1466; 1976.

HERBECK G. Kritische Anmerkungen zum Thema "Kolposkopie und Früherkennung." Frauenarzt 20: 103; 1979.

HERBECK G. Laser-Therapie an der Cervix uteri. Geburtsh Frauenheilk 40: 904; 1980.

HERBECK G. Krebsvorsorge an der Portio – reformbedürftig? Gynäkologische Vorsorge und Frühdiagnostik. Aktuelle Erkenntnisse zur zervikalen Neoplasie. Fortschr Med 97: 481; 1979.

HERBECK G., F. C. MENKEN. Colposcopy in the management of early cervical neoplasia. Endoscopy 9: 234–238; 1977.

HIERSCHE H. D., W. NAGL. Regeneration of secretory epithelium in the human endocervix. Arch Gynecol 229: 83–90; 1980.

HIERSCHE H. D., R. WAGNER. Die Struktur des cervicalen Drüsenfeldes im menschlichen Uterus (eine rasterelektronenmikroskopische Studie). Arch Gynäk 216: 23; 1974.

HIERSCHE H. D., B. BUSCH, K. W. TIETZE, J. INTHRA-PHUVASAK. Funktionelle Morphologie des cervicalen Stroma im menschlichen Uterus. Arch Gynäk 217: 427; 1974.

HILFRICH H. J., P. HOFMANN. Über das Scheidenstumpfrezidiv des Carcinoma in situ der Zervix. Geburtsh Frauenheilk 33: 212–216; 1973.

HILGARTH M. Verläßlichkeit und Fehlbeurteilungsbereiche der zytologischen Tumordiagnostik. Z Allg Med 53: 903; 1977.

HILGARTH M. Die zervikale intraepitheliale Neoplasie. Gynäkol Prax 9: 51–63; 1985.

HILGARTH M., A. GÖPPINGER, A. ROSS, A. PFLEIDERER. Leistungsfähigkeit der kombinierten Krebsvorsorge an der Zervix uteri. Der Frauenarzt 3: 61–62; 1984.

HILGARTH M., W. HARTLEITNER. Krebsfrüherkennung bei der jungen Frau. Fortschr Med 96: 1020–1022; 1978.

HILGARTH M., W. HARTLEITNER. Krebsfrüherkennung bei der jungen Frau. Wann soll Krebsvorsorge beginnen? Fortschr Med 96: 1020; 1978.

HILGARTH M., H. G. HILLEMANNS. Zervixkarzinom: Was leistet die kombinierte Krebsvorsorge? Dtsch Ärztebl 81: 2017–2018; 1984.

HILLEMANNS H. G., M. HILGARTH. Vorsorgeuntersuchung der Organe: Gebärmutterhalskrebs. Verh Dtsch Krebsges 3: 41–48; 1982.

HILLEMANNS H. G., J. E. AYRE, J. M. LE GUERRIER: Die Einwirkung von Steroiden auf Krebsvorstadien an der Cervix. Ein Beitrag zum Problem des Hormonfaktors in der Carcinogenese, kolposkopische, cytologische und histologische Beobachtungen. Arzneimittel Forsch (Drug Research) 14: 784; 1964.

HILLEMANNS H. G., M. HILGARTH. Frühdiagnostische Therapie des Zervixkarzinoms. Diagnostik Intensivmedizin 9: 23–29; 1984.

HILLEMANNS H. G., H. VESTNER. Über eine ambulatorisch durchführbare Gewebsentnahme-Methode zur histologischen Beurteilung von Portioveränderungen. Geburtsh Frauenheilk 16: 931; 1956.

HINSELMANN H. Janusgrün, ein wertvolles Färbemittel in der modernen Kolposkopie. Laboratoriumsblätter Behringwerke 22; 1958.

HINSELMANN H. Die Essigsäureprobe, ein Bestandteil der erweiterten Kolposkopie. Dtsch Med Wschr 63: 40; 1938.

HINSELMANN H. Die Kolposkopie, mit einem Beitrag über die Kolpofotografie. Wuppertal: Girardet, 1954. Cited in Geburtsh Frauenheilk 14: 1063; 1954.

HOFMANN D. Früherkennung und Frühsymptome der weiblichen Genitalkarzinome. Dtsch Med J 22: 269; 1971.

HOFMANN H., H.-G. NEUMANN, G. SEIDENSCHNUR. Probleme der Früherfassung des Zervixkarzinoms II: Modell zur Reihenuntersuchung einer weiblichen Population auf Computerbasis. Arch Geschwulstforsch 40: 362; 1972.

HOHLBEIN R. Die Fluoreszenz-Kolposkopie und Fluoreszenz-Kolpofotografie. Geburtsh Frauenheilk 19: 656; 1959.

HOHLBEIN R., R. KRIMMENAU. Die intracervicale Lokalisation des gesteigert atypischen Epithels und des Microcarcinoms. Geburtsh Frauenheilk 18: 1030; 1958.

HOLTORFF J. Kolposkopische Kriterien der atypischen Umwandlungszone. Geburtsh Frauenheilk 20: 931; 1960.

HOLTORFF J. Kolposkopische und histologische Befunde an der Portio vaginalis beim Trichomonadenbefall der Scheide. Arch Gynäk 195: 59; 1961.

HOLTORFF J., R. KRIMMENAU. Untersuchungen über das kolposkopische und histologische Bild der sog. Trichomonadenvaginitis. Geburtsh Frauenheilk 20: 229; 1960.

HOMOLAR W. Zur Frage der Gebärmutterkrebsvorsorge in der Facharztpraxis. Wien Klin Wschr 85: 236; 1973.

HORCAJO N. Über den Wert der Anwendung eines vasokonstriktorischen Peptids als Zusatzuntersuchung der Kolposkopie. Geburtsh Frauenheilk 36: 388–392; 1976.

HORNSTIEN P. O. Praeneoplasien der Epidermis. Dtsch Ärztebl 27: 1717–1722; 1980.

HUBER H., W. ZECHMANN. Die zervikale Ektopie beim Kind und jungen Mädchen. Geburtsh Frauenheilk 34: 97; 1974.

JAEGER J. Zur Früherkennung der Uteruskarzinome. Fortschr Med 85: 640; 1967.

JAKOB A. Geschichte der Kolposkopie in Argentinien. Proceedings of the First World Congress for Colposcopy and Cervical Pathology, 1973. Molachino Establ. Grafico, S. A. San Martin 540, Rosario, Argentina.

JANISCH H., R. KLEIN, H. KREMER. Die Früherfassung des Gebärmutterhalskrebses – ihre Organisation und Problematik. Geburtsh Frauenheilk 19: 63; 1959.

JENNY J. Die Stellung der Kolposkopie in der gynäkologischen Untersuchung. Personal Communication.

KAISER F., L. MOLTZ. Arbeitsstudie zur Organisation der Erfassung und Behandlung von Vorstufen des Gebärmutterhalskrebses. I. Ärztl Fortbild 67: 92; 1973.

KAMMERLANDER H. Sog. Ovulationshemmer und Vorstadien des Zervixkarzinoms. Ärztliche Praxis 91: 4483; 1972.

KARAGEOSOV I., D. MISCHEV. Kolpitis emphysematosa trichomonalis. Zbl Gynäk 96: 78–84; 1974.

KARAGEOSOV I. CIN bei Frauen unter 25 Jahren. Presented at the Sixth Conference of the Association for the Study of the Uterine Cervix, 1982.

KAUFMANN C. Früherkennung des Collumcarcinoms. Leistungen und Grenzen der Kolposkopie, Cytologie und Histologie. 51. Tagung Dtsch Ges Gynäk Heidelberg 1956. Berlin: Springer; 1957.

KERN G., H. P. BÖTZELEN. Registrierung von zytologischen und kolposkopischen Befunden mit der Handlochkarte. Geburtsh Frauenheilk 19: 871; 1959.

KERN G., W-D. HOFMANN. Häufigkeit und Diagnostik des Kollumkarzinoms. Med Klin 67: 1197; 1972.

KERN G., E. RISSMANN, G. HUND. Die Leistungsfähigkeit der Kolposkopie bei der Frühdiagnostik des Kollumkarzinoms. Arch Gynäk 199: 526; 1964. Cited in Geburtsh Frauenheilk 25: 379; 1965.

KINDERMANN G. Beeinflussung des Zervixepithels durch Ovulationshemmer aus der Sicht des Klinikers und Morphologen. Presented at the First Conference of the Association for the Study of the Uterine Cervix, Wiesbaden, 1972. GBK-Mitteilungsdienst 6: 839; 1973.

KINDERMANN G. Krebsfrüherkennung und operative Gynäkologie. I. Zur Praxis der Vorsorgeuntersuchungen sowie über Auswirkungen auf Krebsdiagnostik und Krebstherapie. Geburtsh Frauenheilk 39: 3; 1979.

KINDERMANN G. Krebsfrüherkennung und operative Gynäkologie. II. Über allgemeine Auswirkungen der Vorsorgeuntersuchung auf die operative Gynäkologie. Geburtsh Frauenheilk 39: 89; 1979.

KIRCHNER H., R. BRAUN. Klinische Bedeutung von Infektionen mit Herpes simplex-Viren. Dtsch Ärztebl 83: 2433–2438; 1986.

KLEMM M., L. KÖHLER, S. GLÜCK, H. D. REICHARDT: Kolposkopische und zytologische Befunde bei 5046 weiblichen Beschäftigten der Chemie-Industrie. Zbl Gynäk 94: 1782; 1972.

KLIMEK R., J. MADEJ. Octrapressin in colposcopy. Oxytocin and its analogues. Cracow 1964; PESp. 115–122.

KOLLER O., T. KOLSTAD. Die Bedeutung des kolposkopischen Gefäßbildes beim Zervixkarzinom. GBK-Mitteilungsdienst 5: 495; 1969.

KOS J., V. I. MIKOLÁŠ, V. LANĚ. Das Bild des terminalen Blutgefäßnetzes auf der karzinomatösen Cervix uteri. Zbl Gynäk 82: 1487; 1960.

KOSS L. G. Dysplasia – a real concept or misnomer? Obstet Gynecol 51: 374–379; 1978.

KOSS L. G. Praekanzeröse Veränderungen des Epithels der Cervix uteri. Session held at the Ninth Workshop for Clinical Cytology, Munich, 1987.

KRIMMENAU R. Kolposkopische Diagnose der Plattenepithelpapillome an der Portio uteri. Geburtsh Frauenheilk 20: 488; 1960.

KRÜGER E. H. Möglichkeiten und Grenzen der Kolpophotographie. Geburtsh Frauenheilk 17: 529; 1957.

KRÜGER E. H. Die heutigen Möglichkeiten und Grenzen bei der klinischen Objektivierung und Dokumentation auffälliger Veränderungen an der Portio uteri vaginalis in ihrer Bedeutung für die Praxis. Habilitationsschrift, Halle, 1960.

KRÜGER E. H. Über die Kolposkopie und die Möglichkeiten ihrer Erlernung. Med Klin 52: 1781; 1957.

KRÜGER E. H. Praktische Kolposkopie. Med Klin 55: 2006, 2053, 2110; 1960.

KRÜGER E. H. Zur Frage der Gewebsentnahme bei suspekter Portio zur Klärung der klinischen Verdachtsdiagnose. Geburtsh Frauenheilk 18: 271; 1958.

KRUPINSKI L., J. MADEJ. Zytologische und kolposkopische Diagnose der dezidualen Ektopie der Zervix. Geburtsh Frauenheilk 41: 474; 1981.

KÜNDEL K., W. BUCHHOLZ, G. JAECKEL. Kolposkopie und Frühveränderungen des Zervixkarzinoms. Geburtsh Frauenheilk 41: 249–324; 1981.

LANĚ V., V. DOHNAL. Ektopie auf der Scheidenschleimhaut. Neoplasma. Academia Scientiarum Slovaca. 8: 433; 1961.

LANĚ V., V. DOHNAL. Kolpohyperplasia cystica im kolposkopischen Bild. Zbl Gynak 85: 419; 1963.

LANG W. Vergleich zwischen Kolposkopie und Zytologie in der Krebsfrüherkennung. Symposium Concerning Exfoliative Cytology, Brussels, 1957. Cited in Geburtsh Frauenheilk 18: 97; 1958.

LANGE J. H. Die Frühdiagnose des Kollumkarzinoms in der gynäkologischen Abteilung einer großstädtischen Poliklinik. Geburtsh Frauenheilk 19: 540; 1959.

LAU H. U. Klassifikation und Stadieneinteilung bösartiger Geschwülste im weiblichen Becken. Arch Geschwulstforsch 39 (4): 370; 1972.

LIMBURG H. Vergleich zwischen Kolposkopie und Zytologie in der Krebsfrüherkennung. Symposium Concerning Exfoliative Cytology, Brussels, 1957. Cited in Geburtsh Frauenheilk 18: 97; 1958.

LIMBURG H. Zur Frühdiagnose des Plattenepithelkarzinoms am Collum uteri. Dtsch Med Wschr 79: 133, 170; 1954.

LIMBURG H. Comparison between cytology and colposcopy in the diagnosis of early cervical carcinoma. Am J Obstet Gynec (St Louis) 75: 1298; 1958.

LINHARTOVÁ A., A. STAFL, V. DOHNAL, J. LEVY. Über die genetische Beziehung zwischen Felderung und Ektopie an der Portio vaginalis uteri. Zbl Allg Pathol 110: 136; 1967.

LINK G. Die vaginale Zytologie, ihre heutigen Wege und Aussichten. Materia medica Nordmark 21: 123; 1969.

LINTHORST G., A. A. HASPELS, R. ANDRIESSE. Der Effekt der morning after Pille auf das Zervixepithel. GBK-Mitteilungsdienst 6: 850; 1973.

LITTMANN H., W. WALZ. Kolpophotographie. Photographie Forschung, No. 5, April 1955.

LÖSCH W. Prophylaxe des Gebärmuttercarcinoms im Frauenbetrieb. Minerva Ginec 23: 89; 1971.

LOTMAR W., H. J. WESPI. Stereo-Kolpophotographie. Geburtsh Frauenheilk 15: 22; 1955.

LUNDSTRÖM P., E. SEGERBRAND. Therapeutische Resultate der kolposkopisch kontrollierten Entnahme von Kollumgewebe bei atypischem Zellabstrich der Frauen im Alter bis zu 35 Jahren. Zbl Gynäk 97: 449; 1975.

LUST J. Die Aufgabe und Rolle der Kolposkopie und Zytologie in der onkologischen Organisation in Budapest. Presented at the Second Conference of the Association for the Study of the Uterine Cervix, Wiesbaden, 1974. Cited in Geburtsh Frauenheilk 34: 998; 1974.

LUST J., G. GYÖRY. Veränderungen des Portioepithels als eine spezielle Nebenwirkung oraler Kontrazeptiva. Arch Gynäk 214: 258; 1973.

MADEJ J. Die Bedeutung der Gefäßveränderungen bei der kolposkopischen Diagnostik der Vor- und Frühstadien des Zervixkarzinoms. Geburtsh Frauenheilk 43: 606–610; 1983.

MADEJ J. Growth patterns of cervical cancer without an intraepithelial stage, so-called monophasic growth. Colposcopy studies. J Obstet Gynecol 93: 746; 1965.

MADEJ J. Die Anwendung der Milchsäurelösung als Kontrastmittel in der erweiterten Kolposkopie. Geburtsh Frauenheilk 22: 1427; 1962.

MADEJ J. Kolposkopisches Bild des Entwicklungsprozesses der Portiopapillomatose. Gynaecologia 162: 119; 1966.

MADEJ J. The angioarchitecture of the subepithelial blood vessels in colposcopically unsuspected portio erythroplakia. Gynaecologia 164: 283; 1967.

MADEJ J. The vascular bed in squamous-cell papilloma of the cervix and its significance for the colposcopical diagnosis of these lesions. Gynaecologia 166: 466; 1968.

MADEJ J. Kolposkopische Differentialdiagnose der Portiopapillomatose. Presented at the Fifth Conference of the Association for the Study of the Uterine Cervix, April 19–23, Wiesbaden, 1980. Geburtsh Frauenheilk 41: 562; 1981.

MADEJ J., K. HANUSZEK. Zur Frage des kolposkopischen Gefäßbildes des Zervixkarzinoms. Zbl Gynäk 100: 1478; 1978.

MADEJ J., K. HANUSZEK. Kolposkopisches Gefäßbild der dezidualen Ektopie (Deziduosis) an der Portio vaginalis uteri. Zbl Gynäk 98: 538; 1976.

MADEJ J., K. HANUSZEK. Über die Entstehung der Ektopie, kolposkopische und kolpophotographische Beobachtungen. Zbl Gynäk 97: 1293; 1975.

MAJEWSKI A. Ergebnisse systematischer periodischer Nachuntersuchungen im Rahmen der Krebsartensuche in Wernigerode. Geburtsh Frauenheilk 18: 496; 1958.

MAJEWSKI A. Die Noradrenalinprobe als neues Hilfsmittel der Kolposkopie. Geburtsh Frauenheilk 20: 983; 1960.

MAJEWSKI A. Klinische Konsequenzen aus dem Modellversuch Wernigerode. GBK-Mitteilungsdienst 5: 539; 1969.

MAJEWSKI A. Die Bedeutung von Kolposkopie und Zytologie im Rahmen der Krebsvorsorgeuntersuchung der Frau. Roundtable discussion, First Conference of the Association for the Study of the Uterine Cervix, Wiesbaden, 1972. GBK-Mitteilungsdienst 6: 866; 1973.

MANESCHG H. Kolposkopische Diagnostik. Ärztl Prax 24; 1972.

MANGER-KOENIG L. v. Erfahrungen mit der Vorsichtsuntersuchung in Hessen. Hess Ärztebl 23: 111; 1962.

MARCHIONNI M., F. CECCHINI. Mosaic white epithelium and other abnormal colposcopic findings: age-related frequency and evolution. Cervix Lower Fem Gen Tract 2: 33–38; 1984.

MARGITAY-BECHT D. Kolposkopische Untersuchungen bei schwangeren und sterilen Frauen. Zbl Gynäk 82: 1193; 1960.

MARSCH F. Früherkennung des Unterleibskrebses der Frau unter besonderer Berücksichtigung der Möglichkeiten des Arztes für Allgemeinmedizin. A

Allgemeinmed Landarzt 11: 577; 1971. Cited in Ärztl Prax 71; 1971.

Martin-Laval J., R. Gajoux. Die Kolposkopie (Klassifizierung von kolposkopischen Befunden, diagnostische und therapeutische Hinweise). Zeiss Informational Publication No. 83, 1975.

Mayer B., U. Nieminnen, S. Timonen. Vergleichende Studie zwischen Kolposkopie, Zytologie und Histologie. GBK-Mitteilungsdienst 5: 475; 1969.

Meisels A. et al. Condylomatöse Veränderungen der Zervix, Vagina und Vulva. Gynäkologie 14: 254–263; 1981.

Meisels A. HPV-bedingte Veränderungen im Genitalbereich. Session at the Ninth International Meeting for Clinical Cytology, Munich, 1987.

Melzer H., K. Schnabel, F. Genau, U. Wendel. Carzinoma cervicis uteri. Gr O Zbl Gynäk 96: 810; 1974.

Menken F. Ein Stereo-Kolpofotoskop zur Registrierung von Oberflächenveränderungem am collum uteri. Zbl Gynäk 76: 22; 1954.

Menken F. Stand der kolposkopischen und douglasskopischen Farbfotografie. Cited in Geburtsh Frauenheilk 14: 1062; 1954.

Menken F. Moderne Aspekte der Kolposkopie. Presented at the First Conference of the Association for the Study of the Uterine Cervix, Wiesbaden, 1972. GBK-Mitteilungsdienst 6: 957; 1973.

Menken F. Zytodiagnostische, kolposkopische und hysteroskopische Befunde bei Langzeitbehandlung mit Neogynon 21. Mediz Mitteilungen Schering 3: 30; 1973.

Menken C. Fotografische Dokumentation in der Kolposkopie. Dtsch Ärztebl 79: 40–41; 1982.

Mestwerdt G. Symposium über Leistung und Grenzen der Kolposkopie, Zytologie und Histologie bei der Früherkennung des gynäkologischen Karzinoms. Cited in Geburtsh Frauenheilk 17: 286; 1957.

Mestwerdt G. Vergleich zwischen Kolposkopie und Zytologie in der Krebsfrüherkennung. Symposium Concerning Exfoliative Cytology, Brussels, 1957. Cited in Geburtsh Frauenheilk 18: 97; 1958.

Mestwerdt G. Las Displasias del cuello uterino. Limitis entre la benignidad y la malignidad. Rev Obstet Genicol 29: 331; 1970.

Mestwerdt G. Prämaligne Dysplasien nach Ovulätionshemmern? Mün Med Wschr 114: 717; 1972.

Mestwerdt G. Die Frühdiagnose des Kollumkarzinoms im Rahmen der Vorsorge. Hamburger Ärztebl 338; 1976.

Mestwerdt G. Die Rolle der Kolposkopie im Rahmen der Krebsvorsorge. Der Kassenarzt 17 (10); 1977.

Meyberg J., W. Soergel. Frühdiagnostik des Gebärmutterhalskrebses durch Kolposkopie und Zytologie. Ärztl Prax 12; 1961.

Michalzik K. Zur Genese des Plattenepithelkarzinoms der Portio. Geburtsh Frauenheilk 18: 479; 1958.

Michalzik K. Ergebnisse 10jähriger Cytodiagnostik in der Frauenklinik unter Berücksichtigung kolposkopischer Befunde. Arch Gynäk 218: 149; 1975.

Möbius G. Zum biologischen Verhalten des Carcinoma in situ der Cervix uteri. Zbl Allg Pathol Pathol Anat 121: 397; 1977.

Moll R., D. Schlüter. Kolposkopie – heute noch aktuell? Dtsch Ärztebl 72: 253; 1975.

Moll R., D. Wagner-Kolb. Kolposkopische, zytologische und histologische Beziehungen (Vortrag auf der 1. Arbeitstagung der Arge. Cervix uteri in Wiesbaden 1972). GBK-Mitteilungsdienst 6: 960; 1973.

Mosler W., P. Kaiser, H. Randow. Die abgestufte Behandlung der Vor- und Frühstadien des Zervixkarzinoms. Dtsch Gesundh Wes 25: 2222; 1970.

Muth H. Vergleichende zytologisch-kolposkopische Untersuchungen. Geburtsh Frauenheilk 15: 907; 1955.

Muth H. Über die praktische Verwendbarkeit von Kolposkopie und Zytologie für die Frühdiagnostik des Kollum-Karzinoms. Med Klin 56: 341; 1961.

Muth H. Die Bedeutung der Kolposkopie und Zytologie für die Frühdiagnostik des Kollum-Karzinoms. Med Welt 16 (NF): 2413; 1965.

Naujoks H. Diagnostische Probleme der Früherkennung. Gynäkologie 1: 166; 1969.

Naujoks H. Zytologie und Kolposkopie – eine kritische Bestandsaufnahme. Arch Gynecol 232: 91–101; 1981.

Naujoks H., J. Conrad. Der verdächtige zytologische Abstrich. Diagnostik 7: 419; 1974.

Naujoks H., F. Köpf, J. Leber. Präoperative kolposkopisch-zytologische Diagnostik bei zervikaler intraepithelialer Neoplasie (CIN). Geburtsh Frauenheilk 39: 372; 1979.

Naujoks H., G. Leppien, R. Rogosaroff-Fricke. Negativer zytologischer Abstrich bei Carcinoma in situ der Cervix uteri. Geburtsh Frauenheilk. 36: 570; 1976.

Naujoks H., J. Leber, R. Hunke. Zur gezielten kolposkopisch-differentialzytologischen Diagnostik bei zervikaler intraepithelialer Neoplasie (CIN). Geburtsh Frauenheilk. 42: 468–471; 1982.

Nauth H. F. Vulva-Diagnostik. Fortschr Med 100: 422–481; 1982.

Nauth H. F. Vulvadystrophie – konservative Behandlungsmaßnahmen. Dtsch Ärztebl 81: 989–992; 1984.

Navratil E. Symposium über Leistung und Grenzen der Kolposkopie, Zytologie und Histologie bei der Früherkennung des gynäkologischen Karzinoms. Geburtsh Frauenheilk. 17: 288; 1957.

Navratil E. Vergleich zwischen Kolposkopie und Zytologie in der Krebsfrüherkennung. Symposium Concerning Exfoliative Cytology, Brussels, 1957. Cited in Geburtsh Frauenheilk. 18: 97; 1958.

NEUMANN G. Die Kosten der Krebsfrüherkennung. Geburtsh Frauenheilk. 35: 615; 1975.

NEUMANN H.-G., G. SEIDENSCHNUR, H. H. BÜTTNER, G. BADER. Organisation von Mass-Screening-Untersuchungen zur Erfassung der Vor- und Frühstadien des Zervixkarzinoms. Geburtsh Frauenheilk. 85: 893; 1975.

NEUMANN H-G., G. SEIDENSCHNUR, S. SEIDL. Probleme der Früherfassung des Cervixkarzinoms. Arch Geschwulstforsch 39: 264; 1972.

NODA S. Colposcopic differential diagnosis of dysplasia, carcinoma in situ and microinvasive carcinoma of the cervix. Aust NZ J Obstet Gynaecol 21: 37; 1981.

NUÑEZ-MONTIEL J. T., G. GAMERO-LEON, H. GARCIA-GALUE, A. MOLINA, A. LOPEZ, C. GUERRA: Colposcopic aspects of endocervicitis. J Reprod Med 12: 197; 1974.

NUÑEZ-MONTIEL J. T., H. GARCIA-GALUE, A. MOLINA, J. RODRIGUEZ-BARBOZA, G. GAMERO, E. SALAZAR. Study of endocervical polyps using colposcopy. Int J Gynaecol Obstet 9: 105; 1971.

NUÑEZ-MONTIEL J. T., G. GAMERO-LEON, H. GARLUE, J. RODRIGUEZ-BARBOZA, F. WENGER, H. SANCHEZ. Detection of early endocervial carcinoma using colposcopy. Obstet Gynecol 35: 781; 1970.

NUÑEZ-MONTIEL J. T., J. R. RODRIGUEZ-BARBOZA, R. A. MOLINA, G. GAMERO. Colposcopic exploration of the endocervix. Prog Cli Cancer 4: 203; 1970.

OBER K. G. Die Sicherung der durch Suchthese ausgesprochenen Verdachtsdiagnose einer malignen Cervixerkrankung und die daraus resultierenden therapeutischen Folgerungen. Arch Gynäk 207: 317; 1969.

OBER K. G. G. KINDERMANN. Uterus- und Mammakarzinom. Diagnostische und therapeutische Fortschritte. Therapiewoche 21: 672; 1971.

ODELL L. D. What is the place of colposcopy in modern gynecologic practice? J Reprod Med 1: 17; 1968.

ORTIZ R., M. NEWTON. Colposcopy in the management of abnormal cervical smears in pregnancy. Am J Obstet Gynecol 109: 46; 1971.

ORTIZ R., M. NEWTON, P. L. LANGLOIS. Colposcopic biopsy in the diagnosis of carcinoma of the cervix. Obstet Gynecol 34: 303; 1969.

ORTIZ R., L. D. ODELL. Observations on the use of the colposcope for cervical neoplasia. J Reprod Med 4: 97; 1970.

PETERSEN E. E. Condylomata acuminata: harmlose Warzen oder Praecancerosen? Gynecologie 5: 2–3; 1984.

PFLANZ M. Kritik an der Zytologie als Massen-Screening-Verfahren. Fortschr Med 92: 351; 1974.

PFLEIDERER A. Entwicklungsgeschichte der zervikalen, intraepithelialen Neoplasie. Gynäkologie 14: 194–198; 1981.

PLEISSNER K. Erste Erfahrungen in der gynäkologischen Krebsfahndung mit einem Untersuchungswagen. Arch Geschwulstforsch 38: 275; 1971.

PLEISSNER K. Die Erfahrungen des Kreises Arnstadt bei der Aktivierung und Effektivitätssteigerung der gynäkologischen Vorsichtsuntersuchungen. Ärztl Fortbild 65: 1090; 1971.

POPOVIĆ D., B. BERIĆ. Die Rolle der Kolposkopie bei Nachuntersuchungen des behandelten Genitalkarzinoms der Frau. Zbl Gynäk 99: 404; 1977.

RECKEN D. Beobachtungen bei Nachuntersuchungen des atypischen Epithels der Portio. Geburtsh Frauenheilk. 15: 683; 1955.

RIEPER J. P. Intraepithelial carcinoma of uterine cervix with doubtful or beginning invasion. IV. World Congress of Gynecology and Obstetrics. Editorial. Medica Panamericana Buenos Aires 354; 1964.

RIEPER J. P., H. MALDONADO. Beziehung der Epithelgrenze zum Sitz des beginnenden Portiokarzinoms. Arch Gynäk 200: 521; 1965.

ROCHA A. H. Die Differentialdiagnose kolposkopischer Befunde mit der Albothylprobe. Prophyl Zbl Sozialhyg Gesundheitsvors Grenzgebiete 103: 37; 1971.

RUMMEL A. Kolposkopische und zytologische Befunde während und nach Behandlung mit Gestagenen. Geburtsh Frauenheilk. 26: 593; 1966.

RUMMEL H. H. Verlaufskontrolle bei Patientinnen mit suspekter Zytologie (Pap. IIID). Geburtsh Frauenheilk. 37: 521; 1977.

RUMMEL H. H., G. HARTMANN, G. BRÄUNIG. Therapeutische Überlegungen bei Vorstadien und Frühstadien des Zervixkarzinoms. Geburtsh Frauenheilk. 31: 945; 1971.

RYLANDER E. Negative smears in women developing invasive cervical cancer. Acta Obstet Gynecol Scand 56: 115; 1977.

SACHS H. Referat über die 2. Arbeitstagung der "Arbeitsgemeinschaft Cervix uteri." GBK-Mitteilungsdienst 5; 1977.

SACHS H., C. HASCHE. Zur Epidemiologie des Karzinoms der Cervix uteri. Geburtsh Frauenheilk. 34: 921; 1974.

SAUER G., H. LEHN, W. SCHMIDT. Menschliche Zervixtumoren sind monoklonalen Ursprungs. Portion of presentation given at the Seventh Conference of the Association for the Study of the Uterine Cervix, 1984. Gynecol 5 (7): 1–3; 1984.

SCHARNKE H. D., A. JORDE, H. G. PESCHEL, E. SIELAFF. Vergleichende kolposkopische, zytologische und histologische Untersuchungen der Cervix uteri in der Schwangerschaft. Zbl Gynäk 98: 1547; 1976.

SCHAUDE H., P. STOLL. Präkanzerosen der Cervix uteri bei jungen Frauen. Dtsch Ärztebl 76: 3128; 1979.

VOM SCHEIDT R. G. Die kolposkopische Diagnostik in der Allgemeinpraxis. Ärztl Prax 14: 38; 1962.

SCHLAGETTER K. Die kolposkopische und zytologische Differentialdiagnose mit besonderer Berücksichtigung der atypischen Umwandlungszone. Presented at the Third Conference of the Association for the Study of the Uterine Cervix, March 5, 1976, Wiesbaden. Frauenarzt 18: 11; 1977.

SCHMITT A. Colpophotographic demonstration. Cited in Geburtsh Frauenheilk. 14: 86; 1954.

SCHNEIDER A., R. SCHUHMANN, E. M. DE VILLIERS, W. KNAUF, L. GISSMANN. Klinische Bedeutung von humanen Papilloma-Virus(HPV)-Infektionen im unteren Genitaltrakt. Geburtsh Frauenheilk. 46: 261–266; 1968.

SCHRODT U., H. WILKEN. Beitrag zur Krebsartensuche in der Frühschwangerschaft. Zbl Gynäk 95: 1636; 1973.

SCHWARTZ F. W., I. G. BRECHT, H. HOLSTEIN. Trefferquoten beim Screening mit Zytologie und Kolposkopie. Presented at the Fifth Conference of the Association for the Study of the Uterine Cervix, April 19–23, 1980, Wiesbaden. Cited in Geburtsh Frauenheilk. 41: 68; 1981.

SCOTT J., P. BRASS, D. SECKINGER. Colposcopy plus cytology. Am J Obstet Gynecol 103: 925; 1969.

SCOTT J. W., C. A. VENCE. Colposcopy, cytology and biopsy in the office diagnosis of uterine malignancy. Cancer Cytol J 5: 5; 1963.

SEIDENSCHNUR G., H. G. NEUMANN. Erste Erfahrungen mit dem Rostocker Computerprogramm: Früherfassung des Zervixkarzinoms. Z Ärztl Fortbild 67: 1105; 1973.

SEIDL ST. Über Dysplasien und Karzinomentstehung an der Portio vaginalis cervicis. Geburtsh Frauenheilk 28: 1165; 1968.

SEIDL ST. Atypische endozervikale Hyperplasien bei hormoneller Kontrazeption. Geburtsh Frauenheilk. 31: 1006; 1971.

SEIDL ST. Die diagnostische Konisation der Cervix uteri. Gynäk Rdsch 13: 51; 1973.

SEIDL ST. Die suspekte Portio und das diagnostische-therapeutische Vorgehen. Presented at the Second Conference of the Association for the Study of the Uterine Cervix, Wiesbaden 1974. Cited in Geburtsh Frauenheilk. 34: 996; 1974.

SEIDL ST. Die Kolposkopie – eine unterbewertete Methode. Med Trib 13: 33; 1978.

SOOST H. J. Gynäkologische Frühdiagnose des Karzinoms. Therapiewoche 12: 485; 1968.

STAFL A. Cervicography: a new method for cervical cancer detection. Am J Obstet Gynecol 139: 815–825; 1981.

STAFL A., A. LINHARTOVÁ, V. DOHNAL. Das kolposkopische Bild der Felderung und seine Pathogenese. Arch Gynäk 199: 223; 1963.

STAFL A., A. LINHARTOVÁ, V. DOHNAL. Über kolposkopische, histologische und Gefäßbefunde an der krankhaft veränderten Portio. Geburtsh Frauenheilk. 23: 438; 1963.

STAFL A., A. LINHARTOVÁ, V. DOHNAL. Das kolposkopische Bild des Grundes, des papillaren Grundes, der atypischen Umwandlungszone und deren Pathogenese. Arch Gynäk 204: 212; 1967.

STAFL A., R. F. MATTINGLY. Colposcopic diagnosis of cervical neoplasia. Obstet Gynecol 41: 168; 1973.

STEEGMÜLLER H. Symposium über Leistung und Grenzen der Kolposkopie, Zytologie und Histologie bei der Früherkennung des gynäkologischen Karzinoms. Geburtsh Frauenheilk. 17: 290; 1955.

STEEGMÜLLER H. Die Portioerosion und ihre Bedeutung für die Frühdiagnostik des Karzinoms. Dtsch Med Wschr 83: 1861; 1958.

STEFFEN F.-W.. Über die Leistungsfähigkeit der Kolposkopie in der gynäkologischen Sprechstunde. Dtsch Gesundh Wes 24: 1961; 1969.

STEGNER H. E. Über die Ultrastruktur des Zervixepithels, der Dysplasie und des Ca in situ. Presented at the Fourth Conference of the Association for the Study of the Uterine Cervix, Wiesbaden, April 12–15, 1978. Cited in Geburtsh Frauenheilk. 38: 1100; 1978.

STÖCKEL W. Die Kolposkopie, die Diagnose und die Therapie des Portiokarzinoms. Diskussionsbemerkung zu dem Vortrag von TREITE. Zbl Gynäk 64: 1590; 1942.

STOLL P. Über die statistische Erfassung kolposkopischer und zytologischer Befunde in der Gynäkologie. Zbl Gynäk 17: 642; 1960.

STOLL P. Richtlinien für die Aufklärung zur Krebsfrüherkennung. Materia Med Nordmark 16: 361; 1964.

STOLL P. Früherkennung und Früherfassung der gynäkologischen Karzinome in der Sprechstunde. Ärztl Fortbild 381; 1968.

STOLL P. Möglichkeiten der Früherkennung bösartiger Geschwulste in der Praxis (II). Gynäkologische Karzinome. Z Allgemeinmed Landarzt 45: 1101; 1969.

STOLL P. Aufgaben der Krebsvorsorgeuntersuchungen bei der Frau. Fortschr Med 92: 353; 1974.

STOLL P. Zur Bedeutung der Kolposkopie bei der frauenfachärztlichen Untersuchung und bei der Krebsvorsorgeuntersuchung der Frau. Fortschr Med 96: 1670; 1978.

STOLL P., C. GRUMBRECHT. Vorstadien und Frühstadien des Kollumkarzinoms aus klinischer Sicht. Dtsch Ärztebl 69: 2022; 1972.

STOLL P., H. POLLMANN. Erfahrungen mit Albothyl in der gynäkologischen Praxis. Beitrag zur kolposkopischen und zytologischen Kontrolle der Behandlung von Fluor und Portioerosion. Münch Med Wschr 99: 1719; 1957.

SYRJÄNEN K. ET AL: Evolution of human papillomavirus infections in the uterine cervix during a long-term prospective follow-up. Appl Pathol 5: 121–135; 1987.

SZALMAY G., L. JOCHUM, M. KÖLLER. Vergleichende kolposkopische, zytologische und histologische Untersuchungen bei Dysplasien und Carcinomata in situ der Cervix uteri, unter besonderer Berücksichtigung der kolposkopischen Gefäßdiagnose. GBK-Mitteilungsdienst 6: 930; 1973.

TOWNSEND D., D. OSTERGARD, D. MISHELL, F. M. HIROSE. Abnormal Papanicolaou smears, evaluation by colposcopy, biopsies and endocervical curettage. Am J Obstet Gynecol 108: 429; 1970.

ULM R. Zur Klinik des Kollumkarzinoms. Fortschr Med 92: 112; 1974.

VACHA K., M. ROSOL, J. KOPECNY. Präkanzerosen des Gebärmutterhalses bei jungen Frauen. Zbl Gynäk 97: 525; 1975.

VASQUEZ-FERRO E., G. DI PAOLA, M. A. TATTI, J. CARBONARI. Indications for the diagnostic amputation of the uterine cervix. Editorial. Medica Panamer Buenos Aires, 1964.

VERSCHOOF K. J. H. Resultate in der Frühdiagnostik des Zervixkarzinoms bei 6000 Frauen einer gynäkologischen Praxis. Presented at the First Conference of the Association for the Study of the Uterine Cervix, 1972. GBK-Mitteilungsdienst 6: 984–996; 1973.

VERSCHOOF K. J. H. The use of colposcopy in gynaecological practice. Vortrag Symposium on Oncological Gynaecology, Groningen, 1979.

DEVIRGILIIS G. Il ruolo della colposcopia nella pratica ginecologica. Cervix and Lower Female Genital Tract 2: 17–24; 1984.

DEVIRGILIIS G., O. LEOPARDI, G. REMOTTI. Human papillomavirus spread: diffuse cervix-vaginal involvement. Cervix and Lower Female Genital Tract 5: 295–300; 1985.

VÖGE A. Klinische und histologische Beobachtungen am Oberflächenkarzinom und dessen Entwicklungsdauer. Geburtsh Frauenheilk. 13: 970; 1953.

VÖGE A. Kolposkopisch faßbare Portioveränderungen, ausgewertet mit dem Elektronenrechner IBM 650. Geburtsh Frauenheilk. 20: 698; 1960.

WAGNER D., O. FETTIG. Zytologische und histologische Untersuchungen zur atypischen Umwandlungszone. Geburtsh Frauenheilk. 21: 256; 1961.

WAGNER-KOLB D. Über den Wert der Kolposkopie hinsichtlich der Früherkennung des Zervixkarzinoms. Frauenarzt 21: 376; 1980.

WAGNER-KOLB D., A. UMMEN. Langzeitbeobachtungen nach 146 Zervixkonisationen. Geburtsh Frauenheilk. 31: 1022; 1971.

WALKER T. A., W. F. BADEN. Colposcopic and cytologic evaluation of the pregnant cervix. Austin, TX: Texas Medical Association, 1969.

WALZ W. Früherfassung des Portiokarzinoms mit Hilfe der Kolposkopie, Zytologie und Kolpomikroskopie. Cited in Geburtsh Frauenheilk. 15: 949; 1955.

WALZ W. Über die Früherfassung des Portiokarzinoms. Geburtsh Frauenheilk. 18: 243; 1958.

WALZ W. Über die Grenzen der Kolposkopie. Zbl Gynäk 23: 935; 1959.

WALZ W. 16 Jahre klinische Erfahrungen in der Karzinomfrühdiagnose mittels der Kolposkopie, Zytologie und Kolpomikroskopie. GBK-Mitteilungsdienst 5: 544; 1969.

WALZ W. Früherfassung des Genitalkrebses bei Frauen, kritische Betrachtung zum Vorsorgeprogramm in der Bundesrepublik Deutschland. Fortschr Med 96: 1731; 1978.

WASSILEW B. Anwendung der Kolposkopie bei der Untersuchung der Placenta. 4th Conference of the Association for the Study of the Uterine Cervix, Wiesbaden, April 12–15, 1978. Cited in Geburtsh Frauenheilk. 38: 1100; 1978.

WESPI H. J., W. LOTMAR. Fortschritte der Kolpophotographie und ihre Bedeutung. Gynaecologia 137: 282; 1954.

WESPI H. J. Stereo-Kolpophotographie. Geburtsh Frauenheilk. 17: 978; 1957.

WESPI H. J. Kolposkopie und Kolpofotografie. Cited in Geburtsh Frauenheilk. 17: 1051; 1957.

WESPI H. J. Kolpophotographie. Oncologia 11: 66; 1958.

WESPI H. J. Die Rolle der Kolposkopie bei der Diagnose und beim Ausschluß des Zervixkarzinoms. Minerva Ginecol 22: 1148; 1970.

WESPI H. J. Beitrag zu einem Katalog kolposkopischer Elementarbefunde. Presented at the First Conference of the Association for the Study of the Uterine Cervix, Wiesbaden, 1972. GBK-Mitteilungsdienst 6: 912; 1973.

WESPI H. J. Stereo-Kolpofotografie. Presented at the First Conference of the Association for the Study of the Uterine Cervix, 1972. GBK-Mitteilungsdienst 6: 950; 1973.

WESPI H. J. Histologie und Kolposkopie des Vestibulum vaginae. Arch Gynäk 224: 496; 1977.

WESPI H. J. Colposcopic-histologic correlations in the benign acantotic nonglycogenated squamous epithelium of the uterine cervix. Colposcop Gynecol Las Surg 2: 147–158; 1986.

WESPI H. J. Kolposkopische Diagnostik. Gynäkologe 14: 220–228; 1981.

WITTLINGER H., K. HÄNSEL. Erweiterte gynäkologische Vorsorgeuntersuchung und Ausbildung in der Frauenheilkunde. Mün Med Wschr 114: 1561; 1972.

YOUSSES A. F. Entdeckung von Bilharziosis der Cervix uteri durch Routine-Kolposkopie. Geburtsh Frauenheilk. 17: 445; 1957.

ZARDINI E. ET AL. Herpes virus infection of the atypical transformation zone. Cervix and Lower Female Genital Tract 5: 333–335; 1987.

ZINSER H. K. Aussprache zu kolpofotografischen Demonstrationen von A. SCHMITT. Geburtsh Frauenheilk. 14: 86; 1954.

ZINSER H. K. Studien an der gefäßinjizierten Zervix. Geburtsh Frauenheilk. 20: 651; 1960.

ZINSER H. K., G. KERN. Kritische Betrachtungen zur Karzinom-Frühdiagnostik. Geburtsh Frauenheilk. 18: 105; 1958.

ZUR HAUSEN H. Viren in der Ätiologie des menschlichen Genitalkrebses. Med Welt 35: 453–456; 1984.

7: Index